AF701757

BIRD INFIRMARY

EVA ENGHOLM

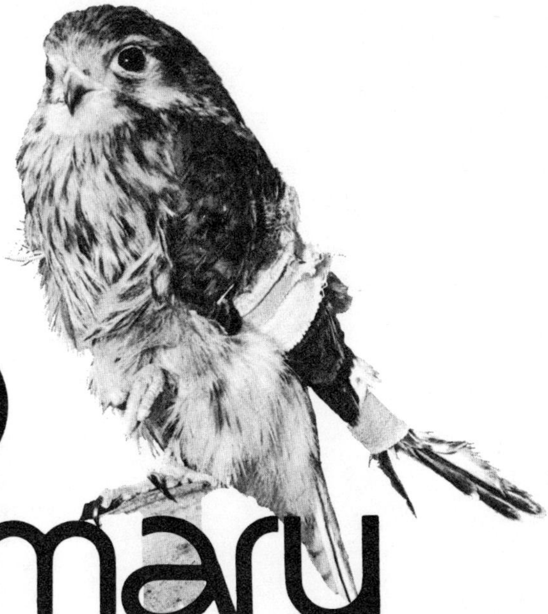

BIRD infirmary

Taplinger Publishing Company New York

First published in the United States in 1973 by
TAPLINGER PUBLISHING CO., INC.
New York, New York

Copyright © 1970 by Eva Engholm
All rights reserved. Printed in the U.S.A.

No part of this book may be reproduced or transmitted in any form or by any means, electronic or mechanical, including photocopy, recording, or any information storage and retrieval system now known or to be invented, without permission in writing from the publisher, except by a reviewer who wishes to quote brief passages in connection with a review written for inclusion in a magazine, newspaper, or broadcast.

Library of Congress Catalog Card Number: 72-6617

ISBN 0-8008-0742-1

CONTENTS

ILLUSTRATIONS

All photographs were taken by Harry Deal, Eastbourne.

AUTHOR'S NOTE

Today to bird-watch or to be 'keen on birds' has become almost a fashion. I distrust such fashions, including the educational ones, as much as I distrust three o'clock conversions. Real love does not grow in shallow soil; its roots are deep, and wherever there is a fashion the charlatan or the moneymaker cashes in. This is dangerous. Since the disaster of the *Torrey Canyon* there has been much publicity, some of it far from helpful to the sufferers.

Long before birds were news, real bird-lovers were working, then as now, with quiet devotion, succouring the starving, soothing pain, saving life where it could be saved, and where not, removing fear with compassionate hands so that the dark sleep might come gently.

I am by profession a teacher of language but the first language I ever learnt was the language of animals and birds. It is a language which is never forgotten and those who speak it recognise one another and as 'ships in the night, greet each other in passing'. May this little book serve as such a greeting.

'And Saint Francis rejoiced with them, and was glad, and marvelled much at so *great a company of birds* and their most beautiful diversity and their good heed and sweet friendliness, for the which cause he devoutly praised their Creator in them.'

The Little Flowers of St. Francis of Assisi.

IN GRATITUDE

TO MY TEACHERS (in order of their appearance!):
THE BIRDS
DOROTHY AND PHYLLIS YGLESIAS
BRENDA MARSAULT
R. B. COMYN, M.R.C.V.S., Veterinary Surgeon, without whose unfailing help, skill and encouragement this book would never have been written.

ACKNOWLEDGEMENTS

I would like to express my heartfelt thanks to my Directors and most especially to my Managing Director and his wife, Mr. and Mrs. J. Schwarz for their interest, understanding and support in all bird-matters; also to Miss Nan Marshall for her selfless, prompt and ever-ready assistance in every variety of bird-emergency, and last, but not least, to Mrs. Stella Gammon for her tireless efforts in cataloguing, checking and retyping the manuscript.

CHAPTER ONE

The Alpha-Early Days

'And does she still dive into the hedge and come out with a bird?' a friend of my youth recently asked a member of my staff. The answer is yes.

I have always maintained that individuals do not change as they get older; they merely get more so, more whatever they were to start with. One of my young friends came into my room the other day—looked around and said, 'You know what? You're getting worse.' Absolutely true; if you like to express it that way. There were four guillemots in my bathroom; a tattered pigeon in my fruit-bowl on the draining-board in the kitchen; a fledgeling thrush in a basket by the fire, and below the eighteenth-century mirror—a monkey. The latter was what the educational psychologist would term a 'deviation'.

One of the best things that ever happened to me was that I did not go to school till I was fourteen. My home education left me hours of freedom to roam the Dorsetshire country-side, and as far back as I can remember, birds were my first love, and provided some of my first heart-breaks. The solitariness of my childhood led me to find rich compensation in the companionableness of 'all God's chillun'. Whereas I frequently found the language of human beings not merely incomprehensible but full of tricks and secret betrayals, the language of creatures was earthy, reliable and made sense; —And like myself the creatures seemed aware of the mysterious, malign and destructive force which used human beings as its instrument, so that I quickly identified myself with its victims and became their passionate protagonist.

I knew every bird's nest within miles of our house, and every egg and fledgeling season brought me repeated agonies. I attempted to guard the nests, and tried to fight off the marauding birds' nesting boys of the district. They were nonplussed, as a hound might be by a kitten, reached mockingly over my head, helped themselves and destroyed, while, once they were out of earshot, I flung myself down on the grass in storms of sobbing and the misery of powerlessness, addressing the distracted parent-birds as my friends, and promising that one day I should avenge them. I even tracked some of the miscreants to their homes and visited their mothers to ask if they would beg their sons to leave the nests alone. As I was very young at the time (I soon learnt the futility of all appeals for mercy) and also small and skinny, wearing garments that were handed on, my appearance can hardly have been confidence-inducing, and from the thresholds of their doorsteps their eyes looked down on me full of a deep suspicion, occasionally most maddeningly tinged with pity. 'Eh, she'm old-fashioned little thing,' said the neighbours, the epithet currently used to designate anything from the mildly unconventional to that on the lunatic fringe.

I learnt the lesson of stillness. Often, when sitting on a stile, the branch of a tree, or on a log with toes in a trickling stream, a robin, a thrush, a blackbird or the member of some unidentified species, would land near or beside me. It would cock its head on one side and the clear, untreacherous eye, full of life, would give me an interested and—it seemed to me—an infinitely understanding look. As I write I poignantly recall the beloved Dorsetshire pinetrees, their resinous fragrance mingling with the mossy smell of bark and ferns, the orange sky behind them melting into purple. We would hold silent converse, the bird and I, until with a cry or a twitter it would flee into the dusk and I slid off my perch feeling comforted and satisfied. I would scuff my way home through the velvety evening, down Coombe Valley, up the stony lane on the right where, if one was lucky one might find a swede dropped off a farm-cart, and down the hill to number 1 Marston Road which was us, above the tin chapel where the local congregationalists foregathered every Sunday to the tinny clanging of the bell. The grating of our rusty iron gate brought my Aunt to the door and to the usual anxious question, 'It's very late; wherever have you been?' I would give the usual half-dazed answer, 'Oh, nowhere in particular.'

I have forgotten how I came by Fluffy, a thrush, the first of a chain of fledgeling blackbirds and thrushes. He grew into a handsome bird of pronounced character. What I remember most clearly is the routine of his daily ablutions. He divided his time between the vegetable garden and the kitchen. To get to the kitchen you had to enter the back door, proceed up a long, stone passage to the large flagged scullery and from thence into the kitchen where Grannie cooked and baked on and in the ancient cooking range. It was always snug in there and under the kitchen table was the shallow enamel bowl of water for our dog. You might meet Fluffy threading his way through the cabbages, housewards bent, with a caterpillar in his beak, or in the stone passage purposefully hopping towards the scullery door.

Once in the kitchen he splashed to his heart's content in the dog's bowl. Then he flitted on to the gleaming fender liberally scattering drops of water over the ginger cat which occupied one corner of it in a state of semi-permanent somnolence. Ginger regarded Fluffy with respect and during the whole of his suave and slumbrous career never attempted to touch any of my birds or even the mice I had at that time. After preening himself dry and picking up a crumb or two from the kitchen table, Fluffy would perform the return journey to the garden, where he was thoroughly acquainted with those crannies furbishing the highest snail-yield. His cheerful banging on his snail-stone would indicate his whereabouts, and in the evening he would plod back into the kitchen for the night. I adored him.

Then my father, on one of his mercurial visits, impressed with my latest protegé, clipped the bird's wings. As he applied the scissors to the struggling bird, he assured me authoritatively, and with his customary groundless optimism, that it would be able to fly well enough to escape danger, yet would not fly away for ever, and surely I did not want that. I believed him though I was hurt by Fluffy's truncated appearance. For some weeks all went well. Fluffy continued his established routine.

Then the moment of anguish came. Fluffy did not return in the evening. I called; no reply. Sick with foreboding I began my search. I knew all his favourite spots, and almost immediately on the compost heap behind the gooseberry bushes, I found the dreaded and recognisable trail of bloodstained feathers. I learnt that lesson too. Never again, cost what it may, would I allow any bird to be restricted in any way whatsoever.

I must truthfully record that this incident only served to intensify my distrust of human pronouncements. The glib assurance had been tragically disproved. I was resolved—as on innumerable previous and subsequent occasions—to pay no heed to the smooth and self-deceiving utterances of human beings. And although Peep-Peeps, Fluffy's successor of the following year, flew into freedom, and eventually successfully reared his family in our garden, he could not expunge from my mind the fate of Fluffy, the beloved.

One day, when I was about eleven or twelve years old, I was horrified to see that the decorators on the roof of the house opposite ours were throwing down the untidy nest of a sparrow which had been located in the ivy beneath the gutter. Knowing that all the nests were inhabited at that time, I rushed across the road, picked up the remains of the nest and collected five blind and naked fledgelings, to the accompaniment of ribald comments from the roof.

I rooted out an old cage, once occupied by a goldfinch which had died at a ripe age. The bird's own nest was useless; I therefore made a hollow in some thick, soft material and placed it, containing the fledgelings, in a corner of the cage. I soon observed how the fledgelings would raise their tiny rumps to excrete over the edge of their 'nest'. Nevertheless inevitably the nest became soiled. My grandmother gave me one of her old red flannel petticoats, and this I cut up into little blankets to make fresh nests for my birds. Thereafter there was always a row of gay red tatters breezily bobbing on the clothes-line.

Knowing nothing, but confronted with vociferous gaping beaks, I popped in little blobs of bread (and bread *was* bread at that time) soaked in milk, and set to, to provide 'natural food'. I produced worms, which I was forced to chop up as they were too large and long, small slugs and woodlice, and even de-shelled and cut up snails. They were all hungrily received though by no means what the mother would have provided.

However, the family flourished, opened its eyes, gradually covered its nakedness and kept me occupied from 5 a.m. till twilight lulled the palpitating little bodies into sleep. From watching the mother birds I had realised that the babies were fed one scrap at a time, and I presumed in strict rotation! Hence I endeavoured to keep to this pattern, arranging that each fledgeling got a beakful or two every quarter-of-an-hour.

The cage was on the wide inside window-sill of the sunny dressing-room adjacent to the bedroom which I shared with my Aunt and Grandmother. They never raised objections to my dawn activities.

Before long I was greeted by a rush to the cage-door, and with characteristic fluttering of wings five spanking specimens of sparrowhood vied with each other to be first in the queue.

Weeks passed and they began to fly. I allowed them to exercise in the dressing-room. They perched on my arms, my head, my shoulders; soon they came with me into the garden; they followed me everywhere to the amazement of any passer-by who chanced to look through the gate. I never had to do more than call them when it was time to go in.

Their flying became stronger; they ventured slightly further, but they still depended on me for food, though they pecked about a bit on their own. I imagined that in about a fortnight they would gradually become self-supporting, and I looked forward joyfully to their healthy independence. It was not to be. Suddenly one of them began to gape; then another and another. Rhythmically, with closed eyes, they gaped. Gone was their delighted chirping; only silence and the terrible gaping. I was frantic. The first one died; the second; the third; the two strongest held out for a few hours longer. It was a heavy, thundery afternoon, and at about four o'clock the last and the liveliest of them all, pitifully stretched out his neck and died. The swirling rapids of grief engulfed me. My tender-hearted Aunt tried to comfort me; I would have none of it. The black and inscrutable force, the destroyer, had come a step nearer, and nothing could hold it back.

That is the hardest of all lessons to be learnt. I say 'is', because I have not learnt it yet. Love must continue to fight death, and sometimes love will conquer.

So, perhaps, the pattern was set.

CHAPTER TWO

The Tale of Austin Pipper

One Saturday evening I was driving back to College along the Pevensey main road when I saw what looked like a squashed chick ahead of me; at the same time I became aware of something struggling against the slightly raised grass verge on my right. There was a considerable stream of traffic, and I was on a curve. I did my best in what I recognised as an avian emergency and drew up. There was a screech of brakes from the fast driver in the Triumph Herald behind me, and an infuriated shout of 'You stupid cow; what the hell d'you think you're doing?' I got out of my ancient Morris, and a ball of fluff on matchsticks swerved madly into the centre of the road. A heavy cement lorry from the cement and gravel works was approaching; I raised a feeble hand and dived for the ball of fluff. There was a lot of noise, and the red face of the lorry-driver appeared above me. 'I'm terribly sorry,' I said, while a sports car whirled past me on the wrong side. Suddenly the driver's face relaxed into a grin. He had spotted what I held in my hand. He saluted, and put the lorry into gear. 'Thank you,' I yelled. As I gazed after the vanishing lorry the words 'Pipper's cement' sank into my befuddled consciousness, later to be associated with the make of the lorry—an Austin. The bonnet had been near enough to eliminate any possibility of error!

I got into the car and looked at what I held in my hand, a peewit chick. A flood of memories engulfed me, and I was whisked back through the years to my student days in Cambridge, seeing outside the wrought-iron gates of Old Hall, the immensely tall and high-shouldered figure of our Principal, Pernel Strachey, the sister of Lytton, and one of the most distinguished scholar-principals of Newnham, towering above the ridiculous little chick I was exercising in the drive. It ran towards her, and I can only remember the gentle smile as she formed some kindly question, while I gathered up the absurd scrap and went back to my room to replace it in the hat-box on its little blanket and give it a supper of succulent worms scraped from beneath the dons' rockery. It had a tragic end after unimpeded progress. Always afraid it might catch cold I placed the hatbox near the fire, as often before, while I went to a tutorial. On my return the hatbox was empty and no eager cheeping greeted me. Then to my horror I caught sight of a fried peewit inside the fender. The pathetic little victim had scrambled out of his box (I had not realised to what extent he had grown up) and had fallen into the fender which was one of the old iron overhanging ones. He had not been able to manipulate the overhang and I came back too late. Sitting in my car, on the Pevensey Road, I felt again the sick feeling of inconsolability of that long-past scene. I must not fail this time. I placed the chick in a box I happened to have in the car and put it on the seat beside me. My collie (whose experience was long and varied) perked up his ears and sniffed, then sank down on the back seat, thankful that this time he was not required to share it with some blood-stained or spiky stranger.

As soon as I got to College I thought of the bird's food. I put the chick on a towel on the couch and tried to feed it a few crumbs of digestive biscuit and a little of the yolk of a hard-boiled egg. No success. I went out and scratched up a few worms. I tried again. Nothing happened. Then I accidentally dropped a worm on the towel, and like lightning the chick's beak darted down and the worm had gone. 'Cheep,' said the chick; and cocked a bright eye at the same spot on the towel. I dropped another worm. It went the same way as the first, and I remembered with relief that, of course, like all chicks, peewit chicks were self-feeding. No need to hand-feed with a paint-brush or eyebrow-tweezers as with other fledgelings. After it had eaten a good supper I put the chick in a nest of cotton-wool in a basket, on its side, my bird's hot-water bottle (a child's cot bottle) under the cotton-wool, and a towel to shroud the basket. It fell asleep. I had my supper, bathed, inspected the basket where all seemed serene, and retired to bed.

About midnight I woke up to piercing cheeps from the kitchen, whither I sleepily padded. There was Austin Pipper (now christened in my mind) forlornly swaying on his matchsticks in front of his basket. Aha, I thought, fresh hot-water bottle required. I filled the bottle with water from the hot-water tap, held it to my cheek, replaced it under the cotton-wool in the basket, noted that Austin Pipper's droppings were satisfactory, and put him back into his little cotton-wool hollow. He snuggled in, and I returned to bed, making a mental note, that his bottle would need refilling at 4 a.m. I switched off the light and likewise snuggled in. To my dismay, after a brief and silent ten minutes, agitated cheeps again issued from the kitchen. Rather bothered and apprehensive I returned to the peewit scene. Austin Pipper had emerged once more. I felt around the basket, all seemed in order; bottle warm, temperature right. Night starvation perhaps. A worm? No thank you. I took him into my cupped hands. He took a fleeting glance over the side, telescoped his neck into his shoulders, shut his eyes and went to sleep. I waited a minute or two and then gently replaced him in the basket. He shot out at once and repeated this frustrating procedure several times. I was feeling ghastly sleepy myself. One thing was unmistakably clear. Every time I held him in my hand, he went to sleep without a second's ado. Whether it was the blood heat, feeling of security or whatever; the hands did the trick. 'Very well,' I thought desperately. 'Veree well.' And took him with me, in my hand, to bed. I piled up my pillows, with my right hand, while holding the slumbering Austin Pipper in my left. (He was *very* small, like a butterfly almost.) Finally I clambered awkwardly into my own roost, and turned out the light. If I were suffering from heart trouble, I told myself, I should have to sleep like this, more or less sitting up, propped by pillows. On the other hand, I was mercifully not suffering from heart trouble, and the required adjustments struck me as peculiarly distasteful. I *did* happen to suffer from the after effects of a serious car accident in Africa, and, therefore, normally slept flat, preferably on a very stiff mattress with only a token pillow.

Well, there I was, upright in the dark, with a peewit chick in my left hand. It was clear that Austin Pipper was content. It was equally clear to me, that I was not.

Somewhere at the back of my mind, there floated something or other that I had read. I remembered that when I read it, I had been deeply impressed, and had said to myself 'to be stored for future use, because you never know'. It was about a sparrow that someone had picked up during or after an air-raid in the war. *Sold for a farthing,** that was it. And I had wondered how on *earth* one could have a baby sparrow in one's bed without—at the very least—squashing it.

I had the tale in my book-shelf. I switched on the light, and hoisted myself (holding Austin Pipper of course) out of bed and fetched the precious document. 'In an old fur glove,' I read. An old fur glove? I had no such glove, but—I went to a drawer and fished around. Eureka! The very thing, a hairy angora close-fitting hat bought at Woolworth's (I never wear a hat) against a Teachers' Conference. I turned it inside out and placed my semi-open hand, containing Austin Pipper inside this cocoon. I retired once more to my bed. I do not remember anything very diagramatically after that. I know I thought 'Whatever would happen if, in my sleep I closed my hand. That would be murder. And what about turning over?' All I know is that in the green and sticky dawn both Pipper and I were alive. Pipper very much so, signalling his interest in worms. I tottered into the park with a jar and a trowel, leaving Pipper, satisfied now, in his original basket. He had a good 'little breakfast' according to French standards and relapsed into repose, while somewhat chilled I made a cup of tea, and contemplated the bleary-eyed future.

I am a teacher, so lessons have to be prepared, taught and corrected. I am also Principal of a Language College, so correspondence has to be attended to, and student-problems dealt with.

* *Sold for a farthing,* an enchanting story by Clare Kipps, 1953. Frederick Muller Ltd.

That day I brought Austin Pipper's basket into my bed-sitting room and put it in front of the fire. I placed him inside the hairy hat (as per nocturnal adventure) on the little hot-water bottle inside the basket on its side. During the day-time this arrangement kept him quiet. I fed him frequently on worms and appealed to the students to undertake worming parties. I promised an issue of free jam-jars for these rustic excursions. The students were willing but urbanised and ineffective. There were even the under-privileged—in fairness it must be said from tropical countries—who had never seen a worm, which hindered their efficiency.

In the meantime I read up plovers in all my bird-books. As usual they were less than useless. Scrupulously 'scientific' and 'ornithological' as they are, not one shred of practical information did they give.* My burning questions were (1) What are the sleeping habits of peewit chicks? (2) What do they *do* during the day; what is their main food and above all *how much* do they eat and need? (3) How long before they are able to fend for themselves?

Also, let it be said at once, I am allergic to the indexing in bird-books. You want to know about a peewit and you start off with 'Plover, American golden'. Laboriously you get round to Lapwing and wade through a great deal of ponderous descriptive stuff to what they eat. 'The Lapwing is useful, destroying more wireworms, tipuled and lepidopterous larvae, than carnivorous insects and worms ...!' Despairingly I looked at Austin Pipper who in his turn was looking enquiringly at me presumably anticipating his tipuled larvae, whatever they were. In another book I found the headings, 'Plumage (there was nothing about a chick, of course); structure; movement; voice; field marks; flocking; habitat; range and status.' Nothing about food or anything else relevant to my problem.

It was a dry summer, and worms were getting scarce. I had supplemented these with tiny shreds of raw beef, but this did not go down very well.

* It is, of course, not the purpose of the traditional bird books to provide such information. They are written for those who wish to identify birds not for those trying to help them in sickness or distress.

Recently I had made the acquaintance of Mrs. Marsault, who, with her husband, had her own flourishing birds' hospital in Exmouth. During my visit she had mentioned maggots, and that these were on occasion preferable to mealworms. I thought that mealworms were too large and tough for Austin Pipper, but I might try maggots.

Not having experienced the kind of protected and sheltered childhood so much advocated by many of the educational psychologists of today, I had never had the opportunity to grow up squeamish, but I did not feel kindly towards maggots. As a child in the country, I used regularly to visit the ginn-traps set for rabbits and to release the agonised victims. I can still recall the nightmarish occasion when standing waist high in bracken, in a dank and mossy clearing in a wood, I *heard* a kind of hissing. I tracked it down, and was frozen into horrified immobility. A rabbit caught in a ginn-trap was a seething mass of maggots in a bloated abdomen, the back legs dangling bloody and uselessly at the end; but the eyes and the head were alive. I now have no memory of what I did, but I do know I shall never forget the horror, the anger and fury at yet another demonstration of man's inhumanity and at the misery of one's own ineffectual helplessness in the face of the terrible need.

I set off round the fishing-tackle shops, where, I was told that supplies of maggots were to be had. The first shop told me maggots were out of season, which conjured up macabre reflections, but I was referred to another shop which apparently encouraged maggots, if not reliably, at least spasmodically when not officially on the menu so to speak. I entered hopefully, and a morose, hard-bitten prawnish-looking man behind the counter said he'd 'go and look'. I had never been in a fishing-tackle shop before, since I do not fish, and during his mysterious absence I examined the 'tackle' and other objects. I was wondering whether the penknives were any sharper than the blunt ones sold in other shops when the hard-bitten prawn returned and announced with a crustacean leer, that maggots were to be had, but as they were not in their prime I could have them for 3d. and where was my container. Here was a new problem.

I had no container and was endeavouring to visualise Austin Pipper's response on being introduced to a middle-aged maggot. In the meantime, no container, no maggots; it was against the health regulations to sell them in a paper bag. It was early closing day. I glanced at my watch; if I was to get back to College to fetch a tin and get back to the shop in time to collect the maggots I would have to be quick and lucky as to parking. Fortunately people were clearing off for their half-day and I just managed to slip inside the shop before lock-up, clutching a Player's Navy Cut tin, trusting that this would meet the case. I carefully watched the prawn's face as I handed him the tin, but it betrayed no emotion. I put down 3d. and received my tin. Keen as a boy scout I rushed back to College and opened the tin. It was half full of cocoons; so that was what past their prime meant. I had not thought of that. However, I picked a maggot out of the revolting perpetual motion in the tin with a pair of eye-brow tweezers and hurried to drop it on Austin's towel. His reaction was gratifying, and several maggots followed the first, after which he shut his eyes signifying repletion.

It was not long before I required a fresh supply of maggots. Confidently grasping the Navy Cut tin I innocently went to the shop on a Thursday (avoiding early closing day) and with somewhat greater assurance than on the previous occasion asked for another six penn'orth. Sorry, no maggots. No maggots? No, they only came in on Tuesdays. Came in? Yes, the cultivators of maggots wouldn't send them before the weekend. Stupefied by the thought that people were busy living, and perhaps sending their sons to Eton, on the cultivation of maggots I dumbly went out of the shop. Next Tuesday seemed a long way off.

I considered Austin's immediate future (and mine!) without maggots and called in at a pet shop. I bought a small container of ants' eggs and a packet of tropical flies which the pet shop man enthusiastically urged upon me. The latter, Austin Pipper rejected out of hand though he loved any flies I caught on the window-pane. I must say their dehydrated legs and pressed look reminded me of instant potatoes and similar unsatisfactory substitutes. I thought Austin Pipper intelligent and produced the ants' eggs. He toyed with these and ate one or two. He also ate a few wood-lice but without gourmandise. I was fully aware, of course, dear reader, that I could have grown my own maggots by hanging a piece of ripe meat out of the window; I was not drawn to this proposition; moreover by the time the cycle would have been complete, I hoped that the original supply would again be under way, and by sending a different student into the fishing-tackle shop every other day, I hoped both to ensure a smooth flow of maggots and to avoid suspicion or unwelcome attention.

In the meanwhile my nocturnal occupation with Austin had come to a blissful end. For five nights I reclined against my pillows, with Austin cupped in my hand inside the angora hat. It felt a kind of boxing glove effect, but I got skilled and could transfer Pipper, hand and glove, in one operation when changing sides. I even changed hands, though not without eliciting indignant cheeping. I even slept. Pipper never did anything else.

On the fifth night, to my surprise, Pipper stood up in my hand, pushing his head against the hairy ceiling. I encouraged him to sit down. Shortly afterwards I felt him scurrying out of my hand and the hat on to the bed. I switched on the light. There he stood, wide awake on the eiderdown. I was perplexed. What new phase was this? After further frustrating experience with the hat I got out of bed, and put Austin in the hat on the rug by the electric fire. (I have lived eleven years in Africa, and my fire is on night and day throughout the year. I would rather be hungry than cold.) To my surprise he did not issue forth from the hat, so incredulously I returned to bed, switched out the light, and awaited developments. There were none.

I had a marvellous night.

From then on Pipper slept on his own.

About a week or so after having acquired him, I went to have coffee with an old friend of mine living nearby in the country. I gave her an enthusiastic vignette of Austin Pipper's character and occupations and mentioned his predilection for

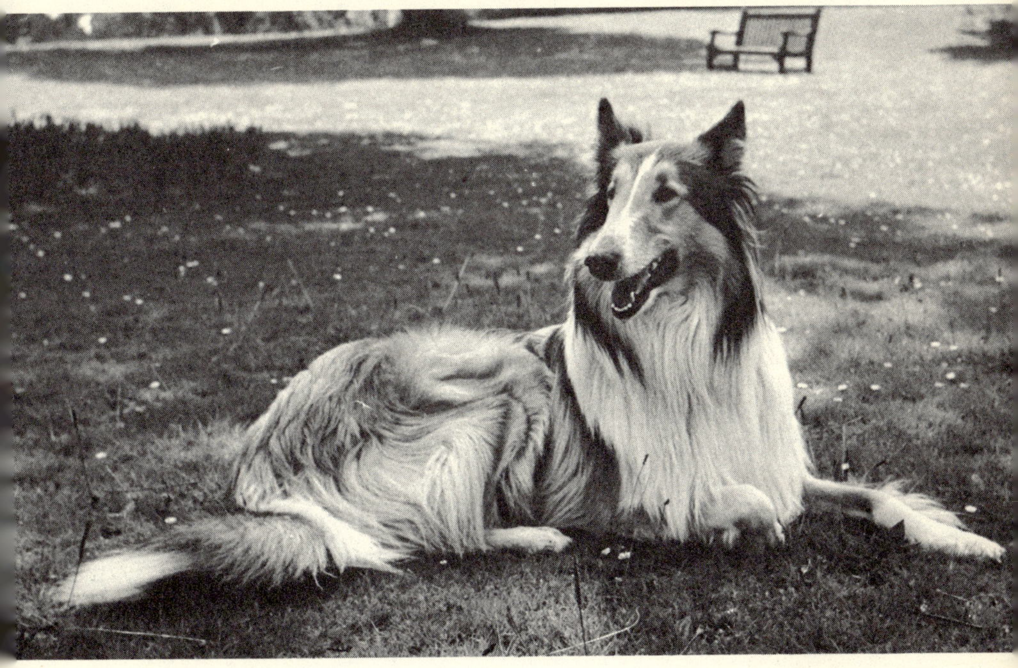

Yum-Yum. 'Fully qualified for canine sainthood' or 'A very parfit, gentil dog'.

A selection of useful baskets and receptacles. Basket with handle on left on top row and with towel draped over it was the home of Moussec, the owl. Extreme right, bottom row, my cat-basket, always in the car to pick up 'cases'. Centre (propped open with a stick) the famous hairy hat that Austin Pipper slept in and which housed the nestful of house-martins.

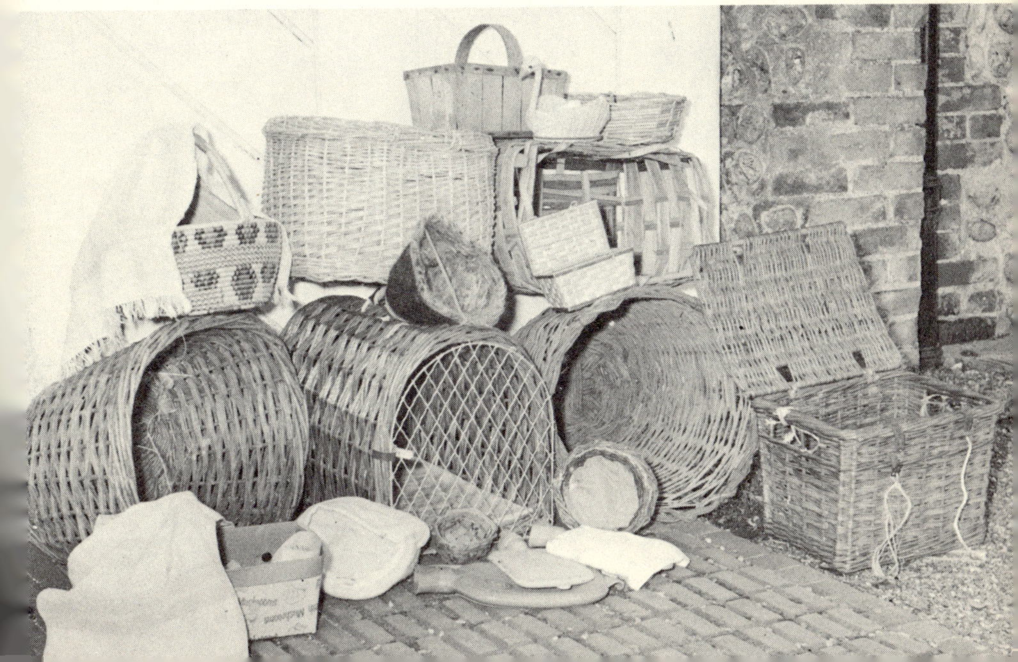

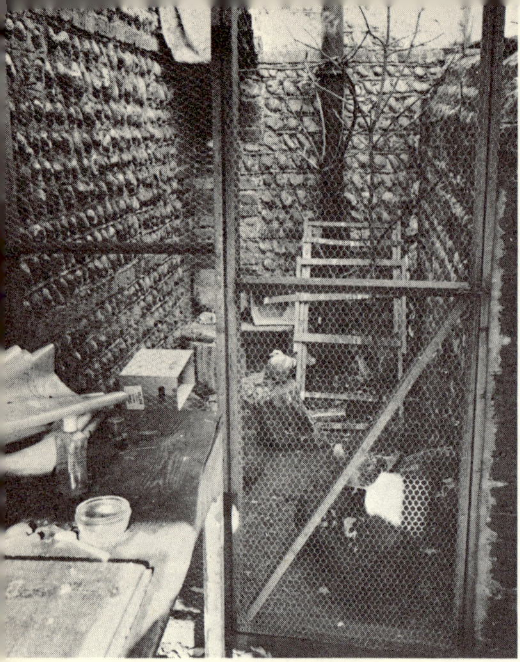

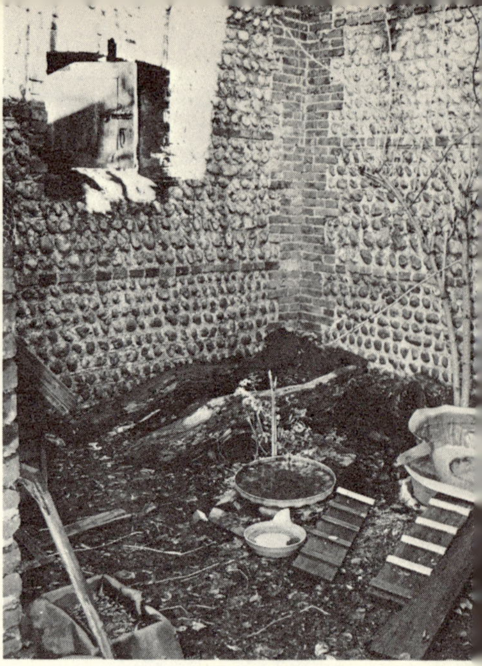

(Left). This shows relation of smaller pen to larger one. (Right). Corner of larger pen showing natural vegetation and variety of 'pools'. Note large-mesh wire covering, admitting small birds and excluding large ones. (This also enables one to release small birds here.)

Convalescent pen with specially constructed cages, to suit different birds. Note left-hand cage with leafy branch inside because it recently housed convalescent tom-tit. (Trousers Ming in background!) Perspex roofing to keep cages dry.

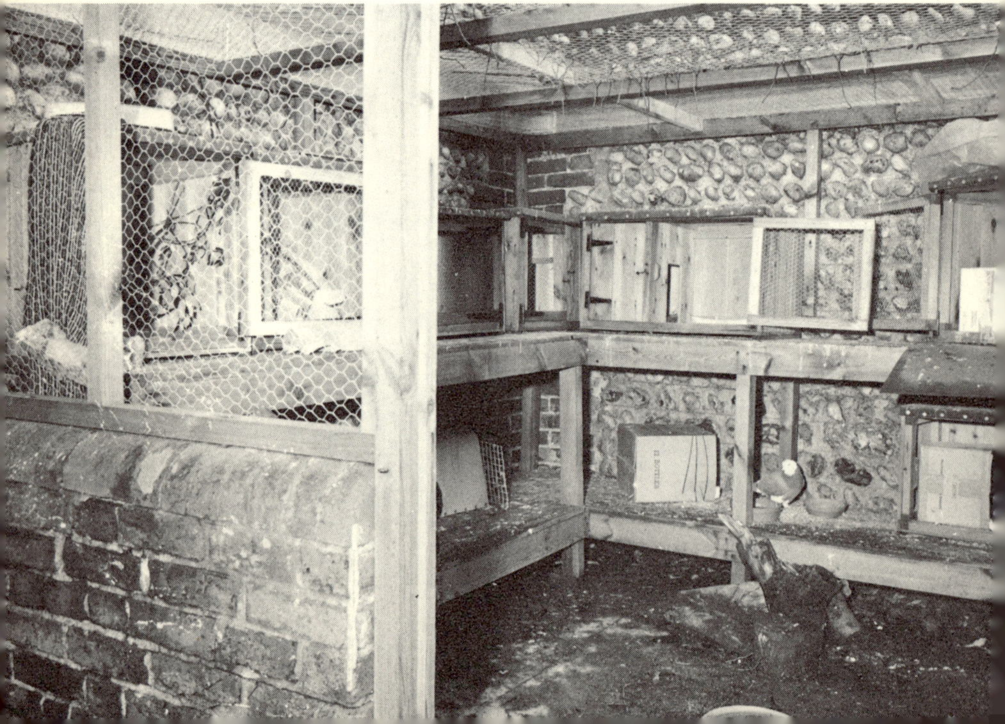

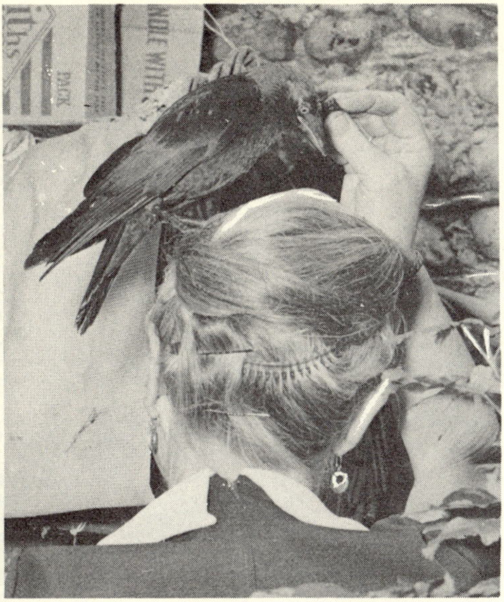

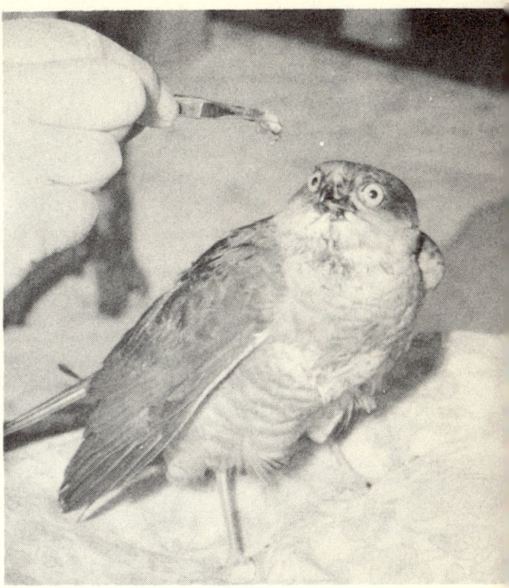

(Left). Jackie Whiskers demonstrating the jackdaw's addiction to mohair seating accommodation.
(Right). Sparrowhawk, found in hospital grounds by a patient. Seen here being fed on my lap.

Hand-feeding liver to a sick coot, later successfully released.

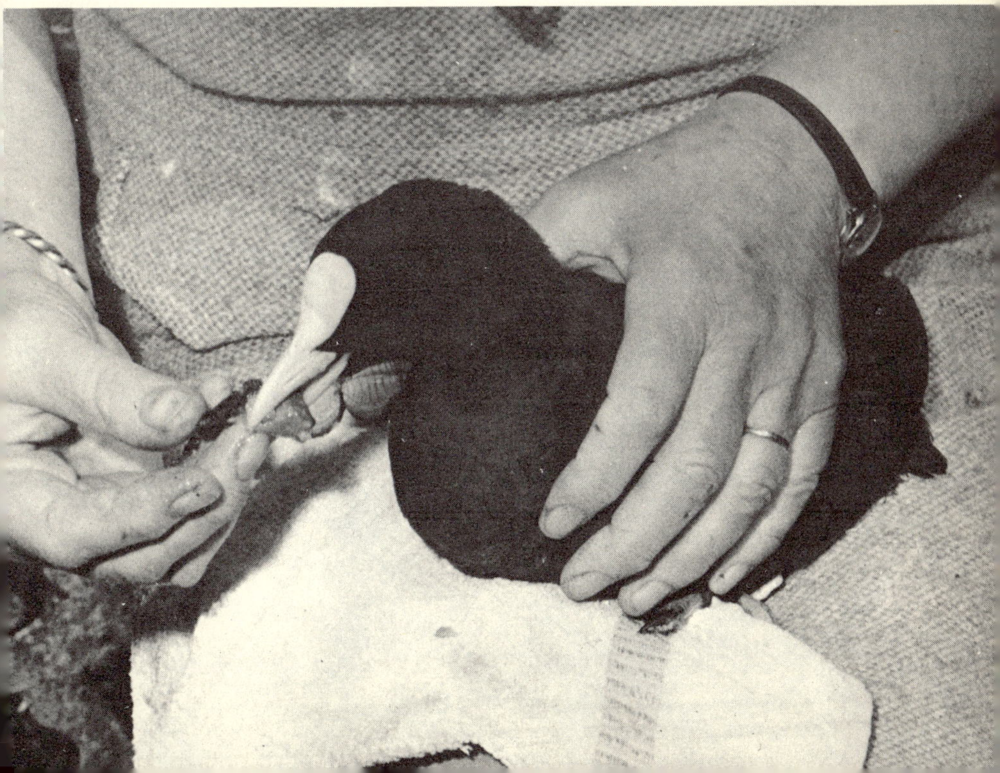

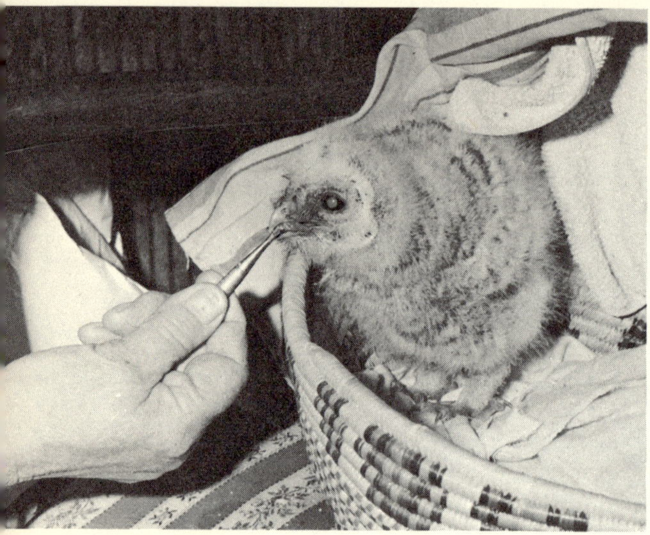

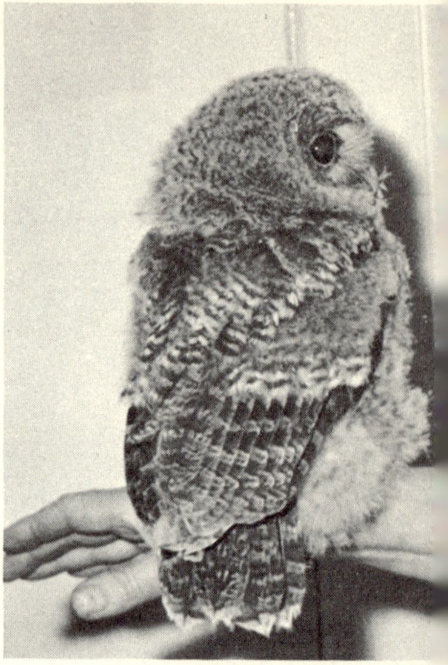

(Left). Mossy Moussec (Baby Tawny Owl) came lurching to the opening under the towel whenever food was proffered on the end of eyebrow-tweezers. (Right). Mossy Moussec, slightly older, liked to perch on my wrist.

(Left). Mossy Moussec on his daytime roost—the top of my door. (Right). Mossy Moussec exercising his wings.

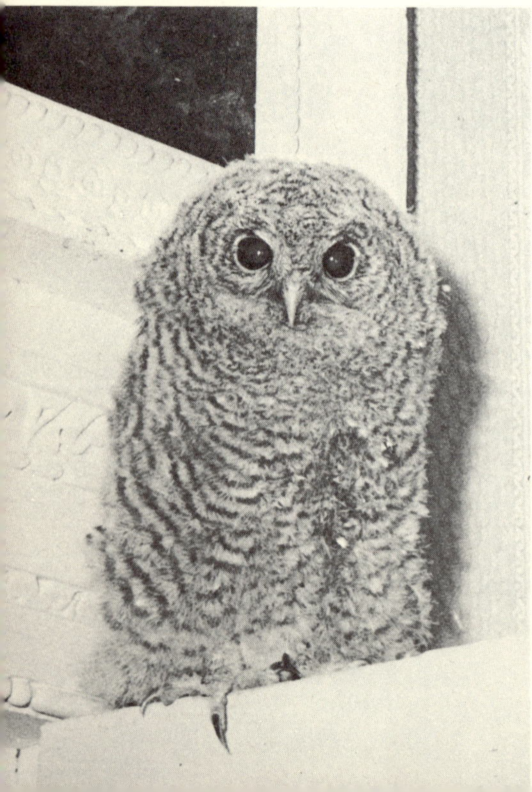

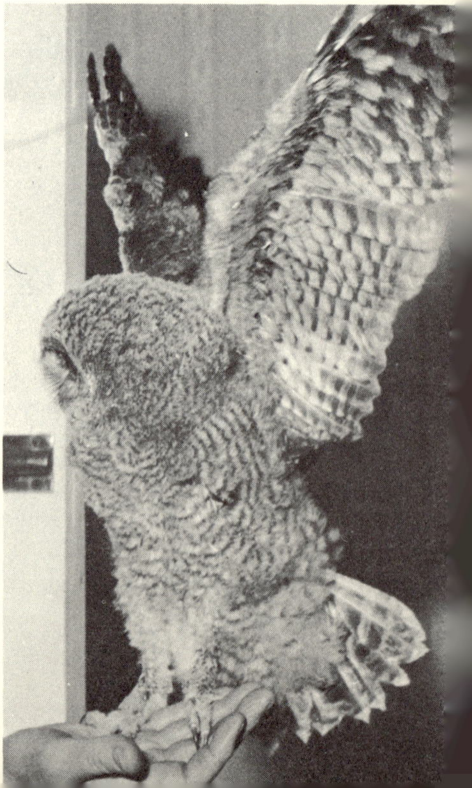

trying to splash water over himself while drinking. She remarked pensively that while on a visit to another friend even further in the country and placed near a stream, they had observed some peewit parents shepherding their chicks to a small bay in the stream, where they had promptly all taken to the water. Greatly intrigued, I could hardly wait to return and to present Pipper with a shallow pyrex dish of water. He paddled at once, shook himself and looked pleased.

It was not long however before it dawned on me that he was looking for something in the water. I set off for Pevensey in the car with a plastic container. Near The Lamb Inn I found a splendid place to fish for all kinds of pondweed; finally I also dredged up a jug of pond-water. I now presented Pipper with pond number two. There was a sizeable shallow iron pan in the stables of the kind one used to put chicken feed into. This I used for the pondweed pond. It was an immediate and unmitigated success. Pipper rootled about and finally stood on one leg in the middle of it. I had placed a flat stone in the pan in case he wanted a little platform, but mostly he ignored this. So he had two ponds; the shallow pyrex pond with clear water for drinking and the pondweed pond for occupational therapy. I had bought a polythene sheet which I had spread along one end of the room under the windows, and on this I had placed the ponds next to each other. I fetched fresh pondweed every other day.

Pipper was growing and showed signs of frustration at his bathing arrangements; the shallow dish was inadequate, the pondweed one too cluttered up. Experimentally I fetched my roasting pan from the gas oven and put that down too. Pipper was delighted and bathed copiously, shaking off the drops in the sun. So the pan stayed where it was and I went to Woolworths and bought another one for my stove.

I used to take the dog on the downs for his daily walk, and frequently passed a dew-pond. Here one afternoon I observed a wriggling mass of tadpoles. Suppose Austin Pipper liked tadpoles; what a feast! And substantial as they were they would surely help to assuage his healthy and increasing appetite. He was by this time consuming, in the course of one day, about

200 maggots, some woodlice, ants' eggs, little shreds of raw beef, also any worms I could get hold of. He had his first feed at about 5 a.m. and the last one at about 7 p.m.

The ants' eggs I had relegated chiefly to fending off night starvation. Pipper still slept by the electric fire at night, but he did not use the hat, though I left it in its usual place, at the foot of the armchair at one end of the hearth-rug. Pipper preferred the rug. Before going to bed I used to spread a towel on the rug, and on this I placed his special night-pond, and scattered a handful of ants' eggs beside it. I then got into bed myself. Sometimes I read, and then I used the angle-poise lamp beside my bed. In this case Pipper lurked in the shadows under the windows, but no sooner was the bedside lamp switched off than he would appear beside the arm-chair. There would be a slight pause while he took his bearings, mainly to see if my collie was safely asleep on *his* rug by the couch. Then he would advance into the glow of light cast by the electric fire. He would place himself right in the middle of the rug, but as close to the fire as he could get, and there he would stand looking at it, like the tiny denizen of some enchanted world; the markings on the fluff of his head and neck made him look as though wearing a neat little cap. At this point I usually fell asleep.

If I woke up round about two in the morning, I would see Austin Pipper busily trotting round his towel picking up ants' eggs. He would then drink delicately out of his night-dish and return to bed. This was a spot a little to one side of the fire at the base of the arm-chair, and the charm of his performance never failed to awe me.

After looking round bright-eyed, he would sink down into a sitting position on his heels, faintly resembling a duckling. Then he would stretch out his neck and *lay* his minute head sideways as though on a pillow, on the rug and go to sleep. When I first saw him do this I could hardly believe my eyes; it is beyond me, to convey the poignancy of the trustfulness of this gesture. I can only say there was something infinitely holy about it, and I felt myself inexpressibly privileged. By this time I had concluded that in natural conditions Pipper would perhaps still have been like a chick under its mother at night, and his head would have been supported by her feathers, while he was enveloped by the security of her warmth and presence. I do not know if this surmise is correct. Pipper woke early in a demanding frame of mind which prohibited any postponement, and this brings me back to the tadpoles.

Although I prepared Pipper's breakfast the night before in order to ease the strain of producing it at 5 a.m., its effect was soon over and by six I was usually driven into the park to look for more substantial offerings. Well-meaning friends who had never lived with a peewit proffered advice of one kind and another—get 'Sluis Insect Food', they said, 'just the job.' This proved to be a complete red herring, not only on this occasion but also on several subsequent occasions when, hard pressed, I thought I would try again. First of all our local pet shops do not stock the special insect-food mixture, because they maintain it goes bad too quickly. The 'universal' mixture they have persuaded me to buy has been an utter failure. No bird has ever touched it, and when I have finally thrown it out on the bird-table to get rid of it, it has been ignored and I have had to clear it away and put it in the dust-bin. Other people have told me they have had great success with this mixture, so clearly there is considerable variety of response to it.

The vision of a supply of fat tadpoles keeping Pipper quiet for some hours was alluring. Accordingly, clad in my old track-suit, I drove off at 6 a.m. one morning to investigate. Grasping an old enamel jug I left the car and walked over the dewy, thyme-scented grass to the dew-pond. The tadpoles were thickly congregated round the edge. I scooped up a dozen or so, thinking this would be a decent haul, and experiencing a fair degree of suspense, I went back to Pipper. I wondered which pond I should empty the tadpoles into; the pondweed pond? Natural setting and all that? Perhaps on this first occasion better in the shallow drinking-water dish, where he could see them, in all their squirming allure. On the other hand he did not like standing or splashing in his drinking-water dish, as he found the Pyrex slippery. Therefore before emptying the tadpoles into it, I went to fetch some gravel to make a steadier base. Then I remembered that weedkiller was used on the gravel of the drive and paths, so I had to make do with a few pebbles I had picked up on the beach.

After these somewhat elaborate preparations I emptied the jug into the dish and stood back. (I had taken care not to handle Pipper; he would have to be released one day and fight his own battles.) Pipper, standing on one leg in the pondweed pond, watched. Then he pattered over to the tadpoles. He disposed of 5 or 6 and remained standing in the middle. I heaved a sigh of relief. Tadpoles were 'on'.

From now on a new early morning ritual was established. Daily at 6 or 6.30 a.m. cosily clad in my old track-suit I issued forth into the fresh and breezy or misty morning. I soon learnt that Pipper enjoyed chasing the tadpoles around the stones, so that I furnished him with yet another special tadpole pond. I may say this was also the last! Sometimes he would eat 25 tadpoles almost at one sitting; sometimes he would eat them at intervals throughout the morning, though he rarely ate one later in the day. In order to make sure I had collected 25 to 30 tadpoles, and also in order to get the ones he liked best (without legs and fairly plump) I took with me on my visits to the dew-pond an ancient and beautiful silver soup-ladle engraved with my grandmother's initials; it had belonged to the silver of her wedding trousseau. It made the perfect instrument for tadpole hunting, as it deftly ladled them out of the little bays in which they clustered together. Thus the operation took only a few minutes, and I could complete the entire expedition in about 35 minutes, giving myself time for a bath before breakfast and a first run-through of College correspondence. Moreover I enjoyed these excursions; the pearly light and the silence, the Downs still free from their crawling burden of ungay tourists. I walked in my sandals along the track, feeling the cool grass between my toes, and savouring the earthy, herb-impregnated atmosphere, while below lay the silky sea, the light from the lightship still flashing on the horizon.

On soft mornings I used to walk along in a kind of sleepy daze sedately accompanied by my approving collie, and taking the absence of any other two-legged creature for granted. I was, therefore, unprepared when, one morning, breasting the little grassy rise on the margin of the pond, I found myself confronting the somewhat consternating spectacle of a very large and brilliantly pink tadpole, in the shape of a naked man in the middle of the weedy pond. As he was not without a degree of embonpoint and was ornamented with what used to be called a handle-bar air-force moustache, I had the eerie feeling he might be turning into a pink frog. It did not occur to me to retreat as I had to get Pipper's breakfast. I therefore proceeded on my ladling operations, along the nearest edge of the pond, with exaggerated leisureliness, while my collie sat down with pricked ears and gazed with interest as the gentleman Neiad got into a pair of off-white shorts on the opposite verge. I believe he also had a towel, but I did not like to appear too inquisitive. He then vanished into the mist. As I returned to the car I could not help wondering, reasonably enough it seemed to me, what someone who under more usual circumstances would surely have been a heavily-suited citizen, was doing in the middle of a rather murky dew-pond at 6 a.m. On the other hand he was every bit as much entitled to ask himself what an elderly schoolmarmish woman in a track-suit was doing at 6 a.m. ladling tadpoles into a battered enamel jug with a silver soup-ladle.

After this somewhat surrealist experience I used to approach the dew-pond more cautiously and with increased savoir-faire.

Three or four weeks passed, and Pipper had grown beautiful luminous feathers. The cap effect was gradually giving place to a little tuft which would develop into the final characteristic crest of the plover. I did not at that time—alas—keep day-to-day records of Pipper's progress, but I do remember that the actual appearance of signs of the crest seemed to me much delayed; so much so that I began to wonder. Pipper's diet remained more or less the same except that when he got tired of beef I gave him little bits of lamb. His consumption of tadpoles was steady but he tended now to concentrate on certain times of the day for his main feeds; breakfast, midday and evening. Every evening before retiring he 'exercised'. This went on for the better part of an hour and unnerved any visitors who might chance to come and see me. This begs the burning question which at once rises to the lips of anyone who hears I have an uncaged bird (or birds) in my room. 'But aren't they dirty? After all they're not house-trained.' First of all let me point out, any bird, or any animal for that matter, is as dirty as its human jailer forces it to be, or as clean as the human being, supposed to be looking after it takes the trouble to let it be. Inevitably all living creatures must excrete. If one's particular love happens to be birds one is singularly fortunate in that the excreta of most birds is dry and practically, if not entirely, odourless, easy to clear away and rarely leaves any traces. Rooks, of course, are splodgy and can be smelly, but so is a cat in a flat, unless properly provided for, not to speak of a human baby.

I do, of course, confine some birds to some sort of cage or pen when necessary for their own safety at certain stages of illness or convalescence, but whenever I first acquire a patient, it always 'lives with me', so that I can make accurate observations at all hours of the day and night. There is no other way in which to be sure that one's observations are either comprehensive or reliable. This is especially true of the night-time. As Len Howard has already proved,* despite the clever non-believers, birds are individuals, and one needs to discover what they are up to at night when they are sick.

Pipper's droppings though moist were fairly neat and certainly not offensive in any way. As I have already mentioned, I had established all Pipper's paraphernalia on a large polythene sheet approximately 15 feet by 5 feet and this he seemed to recognise as his own territory, and the only time he ever left it was occasionally to sun-bathe in a patch of sunlight which came through the other window in the afternoons. He shared the room with my Scots collie, and once or twice Pipper approached his reclining form and examined his paws. After these cursory investigations he ignored him. An acquaintance of mine once said that my collie is the only dog she has ever met, fully qualified for canine sainthood!

Pipper's 'exercise' consisted in dashing up and down, the full length of his polythene sheet. His legs were long and strong,

* In her splendid book *Birds as Individuals*, Len Howard, 1952, Collins.

so that as he sprinted up and down he presented the picture of someone in fanatical training. At first I was worried, thinking he ought to have greater freedom, but how? I had not at that time any outside enclosure. Seeing that he ate well, slept well, and flourished, I accustomed myself to the thought that it was merely normal that he also needed to exercise well. After his exercise he retired to his pondweed pond where he slept, standing on one leg.

End of term was approaching and I was going to move into my cottage. None of the bird-books I consulted indicated at what age a young peewit becomes independent, but I surmised that I must allow six weeks to be on the safe side, and in any case I would have to see Pipper use his wings first. Accordingly I had to brace myself to transferring Pipper and all his gear to the cottage. It is only half an hour's drive but it was murder with Austin Pipper bouncing about in the cat-basket, uttering piercing shrieks. As we passed the spot where I had picked him up, a day-old chick, some weeks before, I could not help but feel that I had learnt a lot.

As soon as I got to the cottage I rapidly laid out his equipment, as near as possible to his previous arrangement: the little Pyrex dish with drinking water, the large pan with deeper water and pondweed, the dish with tadpoles and the roasting-pan for his bath—also his 'night pond'! I put down a tea-towel (without much hope) and his plastic sheet, also his tray of leaf-mould for scratching. It was warm and sunny and as soon as I let him out of his basket he shot to his ponds. He settled down very contentedly, trying (after his supper) to drag off the tea-towel and on this occasion closely inspecting the collie's paws. Owing to the restricted floor space of the cottage, we were all much closer together. I had the electric heater on as usual, so that Pipper came and lay down on the hearth-rug as was his custom.

The next day I was worried, as the sitting-room of the cottage gets no sun till the afternoon while the kitchen at the back is bright with it. I transferred Pipper to the kitchen but he turned round at once and dashed back to his pans, stumbling over the intermediary brick steps. (He was very Donald Duckish, always).

I was much exercised as to what to do for the best, and finally decided to put him in my summerhouse. I had romantically envisaged this imposing acquisition as a kind of little outdoor study, but the day after it was erected, I rescued a young blackbird from the main road, and put him in there and somehow it seemed to have been occupied by birds ever since. It was small and sunny, and before moving Pipper in, I covered the floor with sand and mud and of course put down all the ponds. The fireguard just fitted over the doorway, so that I could hitch back the door, as well as have all the side windows open. So far, Austin Pipper had never made the slightest attempt to leave the ground. As I surveyed this luxurious camping-ground I thought what a good weaning it would be towards a more open-air existence.

It all worked very smoothly and Mr. Austin Pipper expressed his satisfaction with much pecking around, preening and an enormous appetite.

For a week all went well but I thought he was getting restless; he was five weeks old, and I wondered when on earth he would try to fly. He looked beautiful and glossy and robust.

I had staying with me an old student who had written to ask if she could come over from Italy for a short holiday. I was delighted and one leisurely afternoon after we had discovered that we had neither of us been to Battle Abbey, nor seen the spot where William the Conqueror had killed poor Harold, we paid our half-crowns and went on the tour. In the middle of a solemn peroration from the guide, I heard a familiar shriek and said without thinking and louder than I had intended 'That's a peewit.' This caused a few blank looks, but Simonetta had heard it too, and after that, I fear, our interest was diverted from the High Altar to the mediaeval fish-ponds in the field below.

After supper that evening I decided to examine the spot, approaching it from an unofficial angle by scaling a fence and a hedge or two fairly bristling with 'Trespassers will be prosecuted' notices; a further safeguard for Pipper of course, in the event of the fish-ponds offering suitable accommodation.

I was delighted with the whole lay-out. There were moorhens with chicks, a duck with ducklings, and a pair of swans with cygnets. There was a splendid little shore, masses of reeds and bosky bits for cover, and behind these the green fields from whence had come the peewit noises. The whole thing is not far from the sea, with other watery bits in the vicinity. So I said to Simonetta, 'I can't think of anything better than this when the moment comes.'

Next morning we went to get Pipper's fresh pondweed and when I came back I went to the summerhouse to replenish his ponds—No Austin! But nothing was disarranged. I looked everywhere in the garden but there was no trace. I alerted the neighbours but felt forced to conclude he had suddenly made use of his wings. I did not feel very happy but at lunch-time one of my neighbours, two gardens away, came and said, 'Your bird is on our lawn.' Off we went and there was Austin majestically sauntering around looking very pleased with himself. I felt very foxed as to what to do as I didn't want to terrify him by chasing him and anyhow he could clearly fly! He lay down by a little bush for his siesta as usual, and we went back to our cottage, leaving the neighbours to give us any stop press news. By evening he had vanished, and as it was getting dusk I said to Simonetta, 'I just wonder if he'd think of coming back! I'd like to go down the little alley and see.' Well, there he was, sure enough, plodding home! We guided him via the back entrance and he thankfully ate his supper, though he was bursting for water of course. I shut up the summerhouse, relieved to know him safe for the night but the moment, I felt, was ripe.

At 5.15 a.m. next morning, after he'd had his first breakfast at 4.30 a.m. I put him squawking in the cat-basket and stealthily made my way past the 'Trespassers' notices and over the other obstacles. I let him out by the little beach, and he was delighted. I said, 'Goodbye Austin', and went a few steps. Then I turned and saw him going towards the water. I went a few more paces, and turned round again but he had disappeared—into the reeds perhaps.

Next morning I went again at 5.15 a.m. but there was no sign and no shrieks as of a hungry or distressed peewit, so I *hoped* he was all right. He never got very tame (as I did not want this) but he did know me, and had he been in distress I think he would have been around. I called but there was no answer. So that, I thought, is the end of the tale of Mr. Austin Pipper, with apologies to Beatrix Potter, who to this day remains one of my favourite authors.

However, it turned out that it was not quite the end.

Last year I was not at the cottage at peewit-time as I was ill, but this year walking in the recreation ground I noticed a single peewit wheeling over a neighbouring ploughed field. I noticed it because in eight years I had never before seen a peewit in the area.

A little while later, that same afternoon, while working in the garden, a peewit swooped over me. I naturally concluded (correctly or otherwise) that it was the same one, and felt intrigued. I dismissed the inevitable notion that it was Austin Pipper as nonsense. After all, two years had elapsed since his release.

A week or so after this little incident I was again walking my collie round the recreation ground, and this time the lone peewit dive-bombed the collie. That was a good deal more arresting. Then I called, and the peewit came! It walked round me in a semi-circle, and every time I called, it came a step nearer. It was alone. Guilt overwhelmed me, I had released Pipper at the monks' fishponds thinking he would surely make his way to his fellow-peewits in the near vicinity at Pevensey Bay and now here he was alone—not even a wife, on Catsfield recreation ground a mile or two away from his releasing ground. I promised myself that I would bring him titbits.

On subsequent occasions he was always on the paddocks, where the riding-school performed. He always answered my call, but I am ashamed to say I never seemed to manage to organise the titbits. I remembered all right, but the synchronisation in the midst of College life, defeated me. I am writing this on the 20th July, 1968 and the peewits have gone. So has Austin Pipper. Bon voyage, Pipper; happy landings, and thank you for all you have taught me.

CHAPTER THREE

The Tale of Tatty the Cockney Sparrow

'Hullo, I've brought you something.' Ominous words!

A head, wearing a harassed expression on the front, appeared round my door. It belonged to a young friend of mine, once a member of my staff, now teaching immigrant children in North London. As she led a life rather more nomadic than that of the usual nomad, she was generally festooned with an intriguing collection of receptacles originating from all parts of the world. On this occasion I perceived, on one of the lower 'rungs', an open wicker-work basket reminiscent of Madeira or some other Southern port of call. 'What is it?' I asked, peering in. 'Well, I hope it's still alive.' There was a faint flutter among the hay or straw at the bottom, and we emptied out a wisp of sparrow. It half stood, a 'teen-age' hen, still requiring hand-feeding, eager-eyed, and inexpressibly ragged, on the draining-board.

'We tried to feed it, but it hasn't had much.'

While I was rapidly making up some 'Complan', the nearest thing to hand, my visitor explained that a Greek girl had found it in the gutter in Islington and had brought it to school the previous day, a Thursday. It was put in the fume cupboard, with large notices 'Do not open', and 'Do not touch'. They tried to give it some school milk on a school paint-brush, but, I gathered, not very successfully. In the afternoon there was an excursion to the British Museum and on their return, the children had tried to feed the sparrow before leaving school for home. The bird had escaped and they had had to leave it wedged in some cranny behind the pipes of the fume cupboard. The next morning it was fluttering against the window trying to get out, and now after the 'bus and train journey from London, 'she' was on my draining-board. She had had a tough introduction to life with human beings.

In the meanwhile I had proffered 'Complan' on a paint-brush and 'Tatty' as she was inevitably christened, was almost swallowing the paint-brush in her hunger and excitement.

One may never cease to marvel. Here was a tiny scrap of feathers, like the moult off an aged feather duster, galvanised from within by a dynamo that would have done credit to Napoleon. And people say there are no miracles. It is a question of definition and, as D. H. Lawrence has pertinently pointed out, of wonder.

Tatty had several feeds that evening before falling asleep contentedly in a basket on the draining-board. I gave her modest feeds, as after her long fast, I did not want her to overdo things. Nevertheless, as soon as she felt reasonably satisfied, and daylight waned, she fell asleep. Later that evening Matron came to see me, and I showed her the dirty, raggle-taggle blotch in the basket. 'Well, at least that's so small, it won't give much trouble,' she remarked with a note of relief in her voice—but she had reckoned without the Napoleonic dynamo.

Saturday passed off actively but without incident, as Tatty got into her stride. She perched on the edge of her basket, guzzled everything that was offered, with undiscriminating eagerness and watched with keen interest, all that went on in the kitchen. Her appearance called forth ribald comments from mirthful visitors. Small, even for a young under-nourished sparrow she presented a picture of unbelievable and sooty scrappiness. Her apology of a tail consisted of two sad and amputated feathers clinging stickily together at a bizarre angle. The diminutive skull seemed all beak and eyes; eyes alert with life and intelligence. The speed of her movements was positively alarming and should have warned me to be on my guard.

As I have already stated elsewhere, I never confine birds to cages unless absolutely and imperatively necessary, and then only temporarily, for their own safety. I am certain that the actual state of *captivity* is a factor which hinders recovery, whereas the opposite state of *not being confined* is an important, and all too neglected factor, in aiding recovery. I have rarely found a bird which had registered that it was *not* forcibly confined, to abuse this state. They seem to know their territory even if it is no more than a basket, or a perch across a box, and adopt this area as their 'home'. Sometimes they reject the 'refuge' prepared for them and select their own 'home'. In either case I have found this to be satisfactory. Tatty, therefore, queened it on her basket on the draining-board by the kitchen window.

This window, veiled by a net curtain, seems to reassure most birds. The light penetrates; they can enjoy the sunlight, yet owing to the curtain, the panes are not so crystal-clear as to prove disturbing or exciting. Moreover, appreciative students having noted my 'love of flowers' often present me with pot-plants, a variety of 'flower' which I must confess I do not get on with very smoothly. Hence there is often some straggling bit of 'nature'. ('The nature', according to my foreign pupils and in spite of my Herculean efforts I never seem able to persuade them to accept the English version) to lend local colour to the draining-board scene, and this appears to comfort the bird-patients.

Tatty cast rapid glances towards the window but Saturday was a grey day and she was not stimulated to express further curiosity. Lulled into a perilous state of complacency I went to bed in a Browningesque mood of 'all's well with the world'.

At 5 a.m. on Sunday morning I became aware of hearty cheepings from the draining-board. Obediently I roused my reluctant self and crawled into the kitchen. Tatty, unnervingly sprightly at that time of day, waltzed round the edge of her basket, head cocked towards me, expecting sustenance. I started to feed her but she was highly excited and therefore dropped a lot. In order to facilitate my speedy return—as I rosily imagined—to bed, I picked her up to make sure of my target. She ate a delighted beakful or two; then slippery as a small frog she slid through my fingers and hopped on to the narrow ledge which runs along behind the sink-taps and next to the window. There is no real window-ledge, as my 'kitchen' used to be a bathroom, and was converted at my request, for I could not envisage a life without culinary interests. There is, therefore, a slight gap between the ledge and the actual window-panes, which form the one-time bathroom window. I picked Tatty off the ledge and as I was feeding her with brown bread, hard-boiled egg yolk and diluted milk, the thought passed through my drowsy mind, that as Tatty was below the Plimsoll line in sparrow sizes, I had better stuff the gap with newspapers, as she was small enough to fall behind the sink. The thought was no sooner formed, than it became a horrifying reality. Tatty fluttered from my hand, clung for a second to the net curtain and then fell and vanished into the gap. For a minute or two I felt relatively calm. I had on one occasion lost a turquoise ring down this aperture and the caretaker had unscrewed the ledge and retrieved the ring. I had not been present at the operation, but imagined that tiresome though it would be, I would again enlist the caretaker's sympathetic co-operation on Tatty's behalf, and that in the meantime she was safely, though uncomfortably confined in a rectangular space behind the sink. At this point there was a scampering along this rectangle and then a blood-curdling and scuffling fall in the right-hand corner apparently downwards into the bowels of the building. I was frantic. It was 5.30 a.m., the caretaker and his wife were asleep and in any case it was their day off—holy of holies. Mouth dry, and sick at heart I went downstairs to look for tools. As I passed the caretaker's door, his wife came out bearing a desiccated pot-plant. She is a kindly soul whose sympathies are easily aroused, so I blurted out my tale of woe. To my inexpressible relief she fetched her husband who, donning a dressing-gown and armed with a battery of instruments, accompanied me upstairs. Then followed agonising and interminable minutes while the caretaker unscrewed first the ledge, revealing an empty space, terminating at the right-hand corner in a hole round a cluster of pipes. There was no sign of Tatty and no sound. If she had indeed fallen down this hole into some fathomless dungeon in the foundations there was no hope, but worse than that, how would it be possible to go on leading a normal life, washing-up, cooking etc. knowing that walled up below was Tatty, growing feebler with every hour that passed. No, it *could* not be endured. I thought of Edgar Allan Poe, and all the ghastly stories of creatures walled up alive to suffer the slow torture of death from thirst, hunger and suffocation in the lonely dark. It was not to be borne. I begged the caretaker to remove the entire sink and sink cupboard, everything and anything in fact that could be unscrewed. I would pay for the damage. He nobly complied, and in another half an hour the kitchen lay like the ruins of Carthage revealing the bare masonry of the wall, rough floor-boards and debris between the joists but no Tatty, and deathly silence reigned; not a scratch, not a cheep. The caretaker justifiably felt he had done all he could and went to his quarters to look for tea, while I gloomed miserably about the kitchen wreckage. What to do? *Had* Tatty fallen *right* down, or was there the faintest possible hope that she had got caught up or saved herself when she came to the kitchen floor-boards below the sink. They now lay partly bare where the sink had been moved out. As there was no sign of Tatty it seemed almost futile to imagine that she *could* be anywhere further back beneath the boards.

Time was passing and the rising-bell would soon ring. Feeling sicker than ever I went in search of Matron who, having spent years abroad in wartime, often had constructive ideas in emergencies. She came with me and viewed the scene of disaster. 'I should take up the floor-boards' she said calmly.

I dared not fetch the caretaker away from his breakfast, yet every minute counted.

'If I lift up the sink, can you pull away the lino?' Matron said.

Between us this operation was carried out, and fortunately the kitchen floor-boards were loose and of irregular lengths, so that I was able to wrench several out. Debris, odd bricks, dust of ages but no sparrow. Matron had to leave to go to the dining-room; it was nearly breakfast-time.

I was still in my dressing-gown so went to the bathroom to get dressed. Life would have to go on, and the mess cleared up. Without returning to the kitchen I went downstairs to attend to College matters. Then bracing myself, I went back to the kitchen and stood in the doorway surveying the desolate picture it presented. Suddenly I had the feeling of being watched, and turning towards the gas-stove on my right I beheld on the floor beside it a beady eye with a dead-end kid expression gleaming from a fuddle of cobwebs. Tatty had emerged from the gap in the floorboards, presumably and mercifully attracted by the light. Light-headed with joy I instantly determined *no* further accidents. She was hungry of course and slightly chastened too, so she readily allowed herself to be fed and placed in her basket. I then put a towel over the top which I tied down with string.

I rushed downstairs to spread the good news, and the long-suffering caretaker resignedly screwed everything back into place.

I then stuffed up not only the gap behind the sink but positively every crack that might accommodate a pin; after which I removed the towel from Tatty's basket, meeting her perplexed but glittering gaze as I did so. I fed her to the accompaniment of her cheerful chirping commentary, as she hopped in pleasure from her basket on to my thumb and back again.

She had a good meal and even showed signs of somnolence, so leaving her with a sigh of relief to digest it, I applied myself once more to my Sunday routine. An hour later I went to feed Tatty. No sign of her. This time I remained perfectly calm. I *knew* there was not the minutest cranny that I had not filled. Tatty was in the kitchen, but of course, she *was* very small and I had a fair amount of clutter accumulated over eight years in a small space. It included on top of the kitchen cupboard a rich and motley collection of possibly useful bird equipment such as old raspberry punnets, shallow plastic dishes, soft pieces of woolly material; also paint-pots, a toaster which didn't work, and other rejected gear guaranteed to provide the maximum of concealment to a dynamic sparrow activated by the spirit of Columbus. There was a smaller pile in a dark corner by the refrigerator and unanalysed contents in a slatted orange-box which served as my 'vegetable rack'.

I could not bear to throw this away or replace it because it had served as the 'cradle' in a public performance of 'Cradle Song' of sacred memory. The possibilities were therefore extensive and time-consuming. I set to work, and heard a determined scratching. 'So there,' I thought, 'you are.' But where? I stopped moving; the scratching stopped also. I started off again and a few seconds later so did the scratching. I stopped and located the sound in the bottom half of the kitchen cupboard, the doors of which were closed. Mysterious, but clearly Tatty possessed powers reminiscent of Houdini, so I opened the doors and removed everything from within.

No bird, no sound. Flummoxed, I once again went to fetch Matron and explained the ludicrous situation. We went back together to the kitchen. Silence. We waited. Unmistakable scratching in the kitchen cupboard. We were positively *looking* at the scratching; yet it remained disembodied. 'We'd better move the cupboard,' said Matron, although there did not seem to be any room behind it. We duly dismantled everything, and removed a great many curious and more or less interesting objects from the top. Finally we heaved the cupboard from the wall; the first time in eight years. Nothing. Silence. The silence continued. I fetched a stool and Matron sat on it while I perched on a box. We waited, and finally, overcome at the thought of the absurdity of it all we started to giggle. This called forth more scratching, still at the bottom of the kitchen cupboard. The back was in darkness so I fetched a torch and then lay flat on the floor while I shone the torch down the back of the cupboard. At the bottom there was a tiny space between the bottom of the cupboard itself and the floor it stood on, as it had no legs. From within this space apparently issued the scratching. By placing my face on the floor and shining the torch into the space, I eventually located a gleam of eye in the farthest corner. 'Can you give me something to poke round with?' Matron handed me an ancient umbrella. I pushed this in and raked gently round; on the withdrawing end there appeared Tatty, even grimier than when last sighted. I grabbed her, and at this precise moment there was a knock on the kitchen door; without waiting for a reply it opened and one of my most elegant students entered balanced on what at my eye-level I perceived to be delicate stiletto heels. As I hoisted myself into a kneeling position cobwebs and mouse-dirt clinging drippingly to the front of my old pullover a cool voice said, 'Mrs. Engholm, may I introduce my parents?' Visions of the various possible embassies flashed through my mind; I could just see round the kitchen cupboard the aghast expression on Matron's face, while in the near distance moved fragrant figures emanating expensive Paris perfumes. 'I'm *terribly* sorry Ellen,' I said, 'but do you think I could possibly see them a little later?' According to regulations Sunday was supposed to be my free day, and no appointment had been made. I did at least have technical right on my side!

After the student had withdrawn in an aura of dignified incomprehension I said, 'This is positively Tatty's last exploit.' Her feathers were sticking out of my clutched fist, and her rakish little face peered over my knuckles as I was holding her upside down. I deposited her hard-heartedly in a small hamster cage, procured in a hurry to act as a convalescent home for a half-drowned field mouse which had been washed down a gutter in a rain-storm. It had conveniently just come to light amongst the jumble on the top of the cupboard. 'And there you will stay, my girl, till greater maturity teaches you better judgment.' I uttered these words as stonily as I could, though feeling I was criminally confining her to a padded cell. Tatty, quite unabashed, examined her quarters, and flitted into the hamster bedroom and out again. She drank some water from the little dish, shook her feathers, flirted her 'tail' and looked up as much as to say, 'I'm ready for the next step.'

Tatty stayed for several days in 'Hamster House' gay and undefeated, eating heartily, sleeping soundly, and never once attempting to rebel at her constricting environment. At the end of that time she was beginning to pick up a little food herself, so I thought the time had come to put her into the old stable enclosure where Bertie the one-legged pigeon reigned. It has a full-sized branch inside and Tatty could learn to fly properly, and gradually increase her self-feeding. From there too I could release her to join the colony of sparrows which lived around the stable-yard.

And so indeed it came to pass, but not *quite*, for everything which concerned Tatty inevitably took on a special flavour. She was precocious in everything, flew without difficulty, and almost immediately took to feeding herself, but go she would not. She had become attached to Bertie, the pigeon, whose surly reserve she ignored, perching on a twig next to his alighting board and flirting around him with many cheeps and flits of wing; bobbing like a robin and holding interminable and one-sided 'conversations'. Bertie, a hardened old bachelor, would sit regarding her with a morose and pink-rimmed eye, feathers pluffed out in impenetrable unsociability. But she won in the end, and the day came when Bertie welcomed her back from one of her excursions (she left for short outings daily) with a soft cooing, which thereafter was oft repeated. Having gained her point the little wretch acquired a 'friend', a rather timid cock who followed her shyly into the pen and for ever afterwards had the air of excusing himself with head bowed low.

For months Tatty was recognisable in the yard, when not in Bertie's pen, because of her continued bedraggled appearance. She remained a cockney, of stunted size, unquenchable gaiety, and absurd about the tail. She always slept near Bertie and partook of his morning feed. The following summer there came a time when I had to shut the top half of the stable door on account of another inhabitant. Usually Tatty was already roosting inside and was thus shut in with the others; sometimes she was not there and spent the night outside.

It is three years ago now that Tatty, the cockney sparrow fired by the indomitable cockney spirit launched on her colourful career in the one-time seat of a peer of the realm. Happily she is still with us, and though rather more sober in appearance since a moult or two, the inexpressible *joie de vivre* with which she whisks into the stable to share a snack with its various occupants marks her out from among her more stolid and more cautious country cousins.

As we recall our mutual experiences with birds Matron occasionally reminds me, with a rueful smile, 'To think I said "It's so small, at least that won't give you much trouble"!'

CHAPTER FOUR

Jack Devon and Jackie Whiskers

During one of the first summers at the College I had reared an abandoned fledgeling jackdaw, till it had grown into a sturdy specimen of jackdawhood and had joined the jackdaw colony centred in and around the hollow elm at the back gate. His career had been smooth and I only remember his rather endearing habit of sidling along the top of the wooden garden bench when I was sitting reading in the grounds, to preen my hair at the back. He would do this also to specially favoured but unsuspecting visitors who did not always appreciate the privilege. Until he finally forsook human beings for jackdaws he frequently rode on my shoulder or my head; this addiction of jackdaws for mohair seating accommodation can lead to embarrassments. Our jackdaw once caused an awkward moment by taking up his perch on the head of one of our Directors. The bald naturally escaped his attentions as they did not provide the required upholstery.

Then one day, just after morning assembly, as I was hanging my academic insignia on its hook by the window, I saw a jackdaw dragging himself across the lawn with a badly-drooping wing. I alerted my secretary whose extra-mural activities are varied and manifold, and together we approached the weary-looking bird from opposite angles. Weary or not he did not relish being trapped and dived behind the rose-bushes along the front of the House. My secretary bravely followed in her high heels which skidded on the gravel and I guiltily observed that her ensuing fall finished off a pair of sheer nylon stockings. Relying on her imperturbable good temper I called to her to plunge into the rose-bushes by the door while I tried to corner the bewildered bird by driving him towards her. This crude manoeuvre did in fact work at the cost of several bleeding scratches. I was due to teach the advanced group so merely deposited the jackdaw in my little kitchen, nearly always the first repository of an injured bird, and shut the door.

When I returned in 'break' he was nowhere to be seen. I gazed around me and finally observed a beak protruding from underneath the gas-stove. I filled a shallow bowl with water and placed it on the floor near the beak. Immediately the beak advanced on the end of an outstretched neck and plunged into the bowl. The bird drank gratefully, then looked up side-ways with a semi-inquisitive semi-humorous expression and withdrew once more beneath the gas-stove. Owing to limited space I kept my chicken casserole under the gas-stove and in this casserole the jackdaw took refuge, though it involved a crouching position which, one would have thought too excruciatingly uncomfortable to prove relaxing. However, 'the bird knows best' is a pretty good motto and I did not interfere. I had to go and teach again, and when finally I was free, my thoughts turned to its food. The bird's breast-bone had stuck out painfully when I picked him up, and if he drank, there was hope he would eat. Thereafter the wing would need to be attended to. Priority always to reassuring the bird, banishing fear, supplying warmth, water, food, and then seeing to the injury or illness.

I therefore dropped bits of cheese and milky bread near the bowl of water. The beak emerged and disposed of these. I felt great relief. If a bird will drink and eat, fifty per cent of the battle is won.

Now I would need to enlist matron's help and skill. She was infallibly generous about this and before long we were attempting to carry out the instructions hastily requested and received by telephone from Mousehole.

Our first effort at strapping up the wing with adhesive tape was not very good and the jackdaw had very soon made mincemeat of the dressing. Feeling somewhat despondent and inadequate we tried again. As before I held the bird while matron cut and officiated with the adhesive tape. We realised that we had fixed the first tape too near the shoulder whereas it was necessary to heave the wing up by giving it support nearer the tail. This time the wing seemed fixed at a respectable angle and having liberated the bird, who once more retired beneath the gas-stove, we felt better. 'Distract him,' Dorothy Yglesias had said on the telephone. 'Keep his mind off the adhesive tape. Jackdaws like playing with cabbage stalks.' I stole a whole cabbage from the kitchen and extracted a stalk. In the words of the modern educationalist 'it did not provide the necessary stimulus and so failed to elicit the required response' and he strong-mindedly continued to peck at his dressing, much to my alarm. At this point however, owing to pressing culinary necessity I had to open the cupboard under the draining-board which more or less adjoined the gas-stove. It is a simple cupboard with one shelf; hence it merely has a ground floor, and one above. The jackdaw soon perceived the advantage of living on the ground floor, as opposed to crouching in the casserole under the gas-stove. He, therefore, transferred himself, thus also temporarily losing interest in his adhesive tape. Once again we breathed more freely, and I removed the rolling pin and other impedimenta from the ground floor of the cupboard. It was dark inside and warm, and I left the sliding door half closed so that the bird might have the maximum feeling of security.

'What are you going to call him?' Matron had asked, realising his stay would necessarily be a protracted one. 'I don't know,' I replied. 'Why don't you call him Jack Devon?' she said. This suggestion momentarily conjured up the picture of a famous fellow jackdaw at the Mousehole hospital who had been christened Jack Leven since he hailed from the tiny fishing-port of Porthleven. As our jackdaw was indeed a guest in the Duke of Devonshire's house, Jack Devon seemed most appropriate and Jack Devon he became from then on.

For the next week or so Jack Devon lived in the cupboard, his dish of water just outside, and food was put on the floor just inside the cupboard. In himself, Jack Devon appeared to be quite lively, yet he preferred the dark to the light, and he stuck to the obscurity of the cupboard.

I had experienced no difficulty regarding feeding with the jackdaw fledgeling who had placidly eaten everything placed in his beak, but Jack Devon was a different matter. Moreover his gaunt look and bony frame contrasted threateningly with the plump robustness of the baby. 'We must fatten him up,' said matron who is O.C. dining-room arrangements. I was in full agreement but after his first hunger was assuaged, Jack Devon exhibited no pressing interest in his food and evinced a delicate discrimination. He was dainty in his habits and not to be fooled, and under no circumstances would he touch meat, either raw or cooked, beef or mutton, or offal of any kind. So that was that. I seemed to remember the fledgeling had stolidly put away a fair quantity of little shreds of raw beef, but as I did not keep written records at that time I could not swear to this.

At the kitchen cupboard phase of his convalescence Jack Devon ate a mixture of cheese, hardboiled egg, a little, a very little, mixed grain (Swoop), and wholemeal bread. We are able to purchase a special loaf which does seem to have had a nodding acquaintance with wheat somewhere in its earlier existence and does not resemble pulped blotting-paper. It also keeps for several days without exuding livid corpse-like blotches with their accompanying whiff of dank cellars.

As he presumably felt better and more confident, Jack Devon became more active, emerged from the cupboard into the light and pranced lop-sidedly around the kitchen. This exposed him to various hazards and I cast about me for a new modus vivendi more suitable to his developing convalescence.

I thought he would probably appreciate a perch now that his balance had improved, so I got one of those slatted boxes which contain oranges or tomatoes, fastened a perch (a good solid twig about half an inch in diameter) lengthways across the box, put newspaper in the bottom (easy to remove and renew when soiled with droppings) and placed this 'arrangement' on the draining-board. It left a narrow strip of draining-board for crockery, and it enabled Jack Devon to look through the window (slightly veiled by net). It also placed him on a level with the narrow ledge (which had previously very nearly proved fatal to Tatty the sparrow) on which I could put his food, also on newspaper.

Jack Devon was delighted; danced sideways the length of his perch, hopped from the perch to the front edge of the box and back again. (The back edge was against the wall). He loved company, and much appreciated any washing-up that took place under his very beak. He never displaced anything put to drain on the narrow strip below him, and although he occasionally hopped on to one or other of the taps (how he ever managed to remain unmoved even for half-a-minute on the hot water tap remains a mystery), he fortunately never descended into the sink itself.

Jack Devon no longer paid any attention to his dressing; only if some curtailed movement irritated him, he administered a sharp peck and we had to cut off a small bit of the tape which had curled back, and trim an odd feather or two sticking out at an angle. As this did not affect anything we did no more.

In the meanwhile I was forced to study his diet. I added a few sultanas and he would eat one or two. Sometimes he would eat a few woodlice, and a few ants' eggs. He did not like maggots but enjoyed the maggot pupae—in moderate quantities. He would not touch worms but pounced on millipedes and wire-worms. He was also extremely partial to the cherries in cherry cake, or just the odd glacé cherry, and would consume, with relish, a daily square of the saffron-coloured cake provided for tea in the Staffroom and known there as 'the yellow peril'. There was no short supply of this, and a little bread and butter was sometimes acceptable. He thoroughly enjoyed a chocolate button, so that I guiltily allowed him two or—rarely—three a day. He would not touch any vegetables except mashed potato which he loved and on Fridays (fish and chips day) he would welcome a chip or two with keen-eyed enthusiasm, holding the chip in his foot and speedily demolishing it. When I finally made a list of the things he ate, I shuddered, but there he was, as bright as a button, skating round his box uttering squawks of pleasure.

One day, arriving hurriedly in the kitchen and as usual calling a greeting to Jack Devon there was a kind of silent emptiness. One cannot help being in a perpetual state of suspecting the worst when dealing with sick birds. Over and over again a bird apparently well on the way to recovery will inexplicably drop dead or snuff out like a candle and one never learns the answer. Hence a nagging fear is ever-ready at the back of one's mind, and for some seconds I dreaded discovering the lifeless remains of Jack Devon. Then there was a slight movement above my head near the window. I looked up and there was Jack Devon skilfully performing an arabesque with outstretched wing and leg, while clinging with the other leg to an iron hinge not far below the ceiling, protruding in a horizontal curve from a disused skylight type window in the wooden partition between the sink and the rest of the kitchen. In the old bathroom days the lavatory had stood where the sink now was, and the partition had screened it from the bath on the other side. The intervening window at the top of the partition which admitted some natural light and ventilation to the bath was now permanently closed, and its two hinges stuck out at either end of the sink side. Henceforth these hinges were Jack Devon's permanent habitat. He enjoyed flying from one to the other, and we were, of course, very excited to think he had started to fly a little. He would come down to his box-perch to eat and one sunny day when I felt pretty certain that the tape on the wing was too firmly stuck to come off I put a dish of water on the narrow strip beside the box, and soon Jack Devon was bathing ecstatically with the maximum of flop and splash. He spent a happy afternoon preening on his box-perch at the end of which he presented a more debonair appearance.

I continued to ponder his diet, and although I know birds can and do survive on artificial substitutes for their natural food I always feel that whenever natural food can be obtained it should be supplied and aids recovery. As Jack Devon so greatly enjoyed the type of insects found in rotten wood, which I collected from decaying logs with the help of eyebrow-tweezers, I decided to provide him with lumps of this wood which I piled into his box. This was an instant success. He hammered away at the wood, picked out whatever there was to be found, and whisked around showering soggy splinters over the draining-board. He could not have found anything very sustaining in these lumps but they did provide occupation and at least a minute quantity of natural food. I replaced these pieces of wood daily, and when Jack Devon had exhausted their possibilities he retired to his iron hinges, where he also roosted during the night. He now followed a fairly regular routine.

For breakfast about 8 maggot pupae, a sultana, 5 or 6 woodlice, and some mixed grain. At lunch-time two teaspoons of mashed potato (or chips) hardboiled egg, the yolk chiefly, or scrambled egg, perhaps another sultana and any insects I had managed to collect. At supper-time a piece of cake, about two inches square, a glacé cherry, a chocolate drop, chopped peanuts, a bit of apple (nearly always rejected) more cheese, a sultana, woodlice, a few ants' eggs, a bit of hard-boiled yolk of egg.

Nothing about this diet was regular, and I always left food on the ledge between 'meals' so that he could help himself. What Jack Devon valued above all else was variety and he never liked a lot of anything even of something he really enjoyed. His liking for maggot pupae was steady and he ate them daily, but never more than twelve at a time; his average was 6-8. He remained faithful to all the items mentioned but would 'go off' one or the other for a day or two. I always tried him with anything new I thought might appeal; peas for instance. He ate one or two cooked though he was not keen but he did not like them raw. Once or twice at the end of his convalescence he did eat a little cooked beef *fat*—the bit cut off a slice of joint, but no meat, and he preferred fats in other forms, cheese, butter, squashed peanuts.

Jack Devon's appetite was as unpredictable as his likes and dislikes. I would get worried when at the end of a day, I realised he had hardly eaten anything, especially when I thought of what a much smaller bird such as a young blackbird would eat, but then the following day he usually ate heartily (for him, that is) and he never showed any loss of spirit. Finally I gave up worrying and trusted to his own volition.

After breakfast while the washing-up was taking place Jack Devon usually sat upon his hinge looking down in lordly state on the activities in and around the sink. On sunny afternoons he descended for his bath and excavations among the lumps of log. I put out some twigs for him to play with too, and these he sometimes took up to his hinges and dropped them on the heads of visitors who were not aware that there was a bird in the kitchen.

He would sometimes be on his box-perch in the early evening, usually at this time in a pensive mood, and after his evening meal he flew up to his hinge for the night.

His wing grew stronger and Jack Devon began to get into training by repeatedly flying up and down from the box-perch to the hinge; then he extended this exercise into a triangular flight by including the top of the kitchen door when it was open and I was in the kitchen. He appeared to be getting wilder, though always friendly and responsive to those of us who saw him daily. We had gradually removed the dressing till only a small patch remained. Came the day when I thought perhaps he was ready to go. I lowered the top half of the kitchen window (which had only been open a little way so far) till it was on a level with Jack Devon's hinge. Like the Lady of Shalott he looked for the first time (in six weeks), upon the green world outside, as opposed to the imitation. I prayed no curse might fall upon him and watched. Tendrils of jasmine curled into the window; it was still mating time outside. My kitchen has a west window whereas the Jackdaw elm is at the east end of the house. Jack Devon sniffed the air like an ancient war-horse and without more ado he flew out to settle on the creeper outside. He then clambered along the creeper to the corner of the house and flew strongly into the nearby ilex. There he swung on a branch and after a time I left him. Later he had disappeared. I went down to the jackdaw elm and called. To my great joy he appeared but keeping his distance as though to assert his independence. He was easy enough to recognise as, apart from anything else, he still had a patch of adhesive tape on his right wing. He seemed to be flying well, and he was not being attacked by any of the other jackdaws, who having got their mates, perched solemnly in twos around the elm. A day or two later I glimpsed Jack Devon with a companion in tow, and soon after he came to the end of a low branch and presented me with a twig. No bouquet could have pleased me better. For many weeks after that we used to see Jack Devon, adhesive tape intact, scrounging the chipped potatoes I flung on the woodshed roof opposite the elms. For a short while we did not see him but his love of chips kept him a faithful visitor, and he remains recognisable to this day, for in the place of the tape on his once injured wing there is an off-white feather.

Jackie Whiskers was a different proposition, his injury was less severe, hence his stay shorter.

He was brought in one Thursday evening (20th June, 1968), by two students who had found him unable to fly near the tennis courts and trailing his left wing. Having disposed of him at my door they lost all further interest, but I was thankful they had not left him where he was.

He was a half-grown jackdaw, still blue-eyed and a little yellow at the back of his beak, but happily self-feeding. The more yellow the sides of the beak, the more the bird requires hand-feeding. The yellow is an indication of age, and as the yellow recedes, so the beak hardens till the bird starts feeding on its own.

This jackdaw was friendly and bright, also very thin. He had a neat little bunch of whiskers which led to his name. He was pleased to have a drink and a little cheese and hard-boiled yolk of egg. It was nearly dark so it was his normal bed-time and I let him go to sleep in the kitchen on the draining-board, perched on the edge of my wooden fruit-bowl. This fruit-bowl of African hardwood had been a treasured wedding present from a dear friend in Africa. The friend had died and the bowl had been through many vicissitudes, but how greatly the generous-hearted giver would have approved of its present function only I knew.

The next day I broke the news to Matron that we had another wing to strap up on a jackdaw. She had been a great friend of Jack Devon's who always greeted her with pleasure. Hence she approached the job in hand with constructive prejudices. Jackie Whiskers, however, was a good deal smaller than Jack Devon and as slippery as an eel. In fact he removed his strapping no less than eight or nine times, but as this was over a period of about a week and at the end of that he seemed to have control of the wing, we left it, trusting to feeding and resting the wing to do the rest.

In the meantime there was his diet to be attended to! I racked my brains to remember all that I had been through with Jack Devon, and cursed my slap-happy response to Matron's repeated admonitions that if only I would keep records and write down the details this would save a lot of headaches later on. She was right, and later our veterinary surgeon added his gentle but steady reminders so that I did actually keep records of Jackie Whiskers!

They lie before me as I write and the record states that Jackie Whiskers ate only cheese and hard-boiled egg for the first three days plus one or two meal-worms. Then he adored the odd kind of beetle-chrysalis the meal-worms turn into, but would no longer look at a meal-worm. I tried maggots. Jackie Whiskers then entirely rejected cheese, also maggots but adored the maggot pupae and remained faithful to hard-boiled egg.

I tried the various preparations obtainable in pet-shops but he would have none of these. On Wednesday, 26th June, he ate 130 maggot cocoons by 11.15 a.m., having consumed 80 for breakfast. At the end of the day he totalled 176 and 1½ hard-boiled egg-yolks.

The maggot drama had started again. At that time I was fortunate in having an energetic and amused assistant matron who promptly entered into the maggot spirit of the thing. She was, however, even less skilled at dissembling than I was so that the fishing-tackle shop had quickly rumbled the impurity of the motives behind her requests for the standard sixpenn'orth. Nevertheless her admirable researches revealed a second fishing-tackle shop from whence she returned in great excitement one day, triumphantly armed with a tinful of seething contents and announced breathlessly 'D'you know you can buy *four shillings worth*. Some people do.' We began to relax. The man in the second fishing-tackle shop, in no way deceived as to his ingenuous customer's angling propensities, finally broke the thin ice of pretence by growling, 'I knew *you* wasn't no fisherman.' To which she replied, 'But I might be a fisherman's wife.' Thereafter we asked outright for pupae rather than maggots and breathed more freely. Not only Jackie Whiskers but a sick monkey recently rescued from a pet-shop, had developed an appetite for pupae, so that between them and a baby swift which ate the flies hatched from the pupae a considerable number were required daily.

National events soon caused a maggot crisis. The assistant matron returned from her shopping one day and indignantly hurling an empty tin on to the table she said, 'There's a huge notice up—Rail Strike. Sorry, no maggots.'

Jackie Whiskers, who had now graduated to being in the

outside pen, was averaging 200 pupae a day, but in view of the rail strike I was forced to ration him severely which he resented. Having gobbled up the meagre half dozen pupae I had offered him, he would look puzzled and peck sharply at my empty hand. As this did not produce the desired result he would look at me crossly and fly on to my head from whence it was difficult to interest him in any alternative, I would get him on to my hand and he would immediately return to my head. He still ate hard-boiled egg, and after his pupae rationing he reluctantly ate a few wood-lice preferring the hard ones that roll up into balls (a brand almost always rejected by smaller birds, I imagine because rather indigestible). I also supplied the same lumps of insect-harbouring wood as had been given to Jack Devon, but Jackie Whiskers did not know what to do with them. It must be remembered he was not an experienced adult jackdaw as Jack Devon had been. Naturally I tried out everything else that had been a success with Jack Devon, but met with different reactions. Jackie Whiskers was not generally interested in fruit, but would eat a fresh raspberry or two. I have noticed that jackdaws and most members of the crow family seem attracted by red. If I put down a dish of mixed food and it contains a cherry or a raspberry the bird usually goes for the red fruit first.

For the first night or two that Jackie Whiskers was in the outside pen I brought him in; then the next evening I was a little later than usual and found he had already retired in a small cardboard box which had a kind of door, and was placed high up on top of a willow hamper suspended from the roof, for the benefit of larger birds. This part of the pen or 'aviary' has a roof of some plastic material over the wire netting to keep it dry and sheltered from wind and rain. I left Jackie Whiskers in his own selected bedroom and there he slept for the remaining nights he spent with me.

The 'aviary' itself is a wired off part of a much larger enclosure. The latter (situated opposite the jackdaw elm) has high walls on all sides; one or two elder bushes grow in it and it is open to the sky. It used to be used for storing coke. Now birds enter at will to scratch among some rotting logs and to eat the elderberries when these are ripe. A hedgehog was also given sanctuary here but he emigrated.

One evening when I was about to go downstairs to give Jackie Whiskers his supper, I observed from a first floor window, a car arriving at the front door bearing the Corps Diplomatique plate. My right hand was full of maggots, so uttering a warning to Matron, who was just behind me, I tried to escape down the side-staircase only to be waylaid at the foot by a student conducting the distinguished visitor, who had emerged from the car. The latter greeted me charmingly. Returning her greeting with as much eloquence as I could muster in order to keep her eyes from straying from my face, I rapidly transferred Jackie Whisker's maggots into my left hand with what I hoped was a nonchalant gesture, and grasped the soigné beringed one stretched out to me, while Matron cravenly sped down the corridor with averted face and bowed head.

Shortly after Jackie Whiskers was established I was surprised to find him apparently communicating with an adult Jackdaw outside. They cawed to each other, the grown bird marching to and fro on the flat stones at the top of the wall. Jackie Whiskers showed neither agitation nor distress, merely pleasantly excited interest. I dismissed from my mind the notion that his mother might have discovered him, especially as he had been able to feed himself when brought in. Not that this is always a definite sign that the young bird is finally independent and separated from its mother for often the mother still pops the occasional tit-bit into its beak. The adult blackbird or jackdaw urgently followed by an equally large and actually competent youngster greedily screeching for food is a familiar sight.

On 14th July Jackie Whiskers was released. I left the door of his pen open so that he could, if he chose, linger in the larger 'safe' enclosure, before venturing right out into the hazardous universe. I need not have bothered. Five minutes later he was disporting himself in the elm next to the hollow jackdaw elm, cawing and playing the baby wanting to be fed, at, one imagines, the same adult jackdaw who had visited him while he was in the pen. These can only be conclusions, but later on he was going through the same pantomime on the woodshed roof where I had scattered scraps. For a day or two he answered and appeared when called. He was recognisable by his unusually small size, a faint one-sidedness and, of course, by his characteristic approach and mannerisms. He had been very affectionate and readily used to take up a leaning forward position, often wanting what the French appropriately name 'un petit bec'. As I did keep a record of what he ate I give a 'diet sheet' in the appendix. (See Appendix I.) He was an even more modest eater than Jack Devon, except where maggot pupae were concerned. He was still thin when he left but wiry, and exceedingly lively.

CHAPTER FIVE

Speedy and Poppet

(Two sides of the coin)

'I've got something difficult for you,' said the Veterinary Surgeon's voice on the telephone. 'No, don't bother to come down; I'll drop it in for you, round about six-ish on my way to a call.' Apprehensive yet curious, I went to the door when I heard the bell ring. 'It's a young swift,' said the Veterinary Surgeon, holding out a little cardboard box. 'Found on the ground by a visitor in Eastbourne. Good luck!' Then as he dashed to his car, he called over his shoulder, 'I think he should be called Speedy, don't you? A swift must be Speedy.' I would automatically have thought of 'Jonathan' but Speedy turned out to be appropriate enough in the end!

A swift! Insectivorous, and catching its food on the wing! Only two years ago I would never even have dreamt of tackling such a thing, but now I knew the Yglesias sisters had saved several swifts, and I had seen the one that Mrs. Marsault had rescued as a fledgeling, the picture of health and joy of living.

I took the little box upstairs into the bathroom, opened it and lifted out the minute occupant. I was forcibly struck with its resemblance to a bat and I loved bats. The silkiness of its plumage, its strange little feet which tickled as they grasped to cling, and above all the flat yet mousey head with the wide frog-mouth and short pin-like beak. I looked at this mouth-beak and thought, 'will it *ever* open to eat, and if not, what then?' How could I, with my enormous hands and fingers hope to prise open this fragile and Lilliputian beak without doing irreparable damage?

Furthermore the bird's eyes were shut and looked gummed up, and below its beak its thread-like rust-coloured feathers were congealed into a tuft with around them the bare skin of the throat. I did not feel very happy. 'Found on the ground?' Why? How? Where? What had happened? It was fully fledged, and its wing-feathers appeared undamaged. However I had no time to brood. I was due to take a student supper-picnic on Birling Gap beach. I tried to feed it a little glucose and milk from a paint-brush (no good) and then from a plastic spoon. Perhaps a little dribbled in, but the outlook was not reassuring. I placed the little creature on the warm cot-bottle in a basket by the radiator in the bathroom. The basket was about nine inches deep. I put a towel over the top and rushed off to the picnic, having first begged Matron to telephone Mrs. Marsault for advice.

On my return at about 9.30 p.m., reeking of wood-smoke and sausages, I called at the surgery to find out from Matron what news there was from Mrs. Marsault. Matron had carefully written down the details, the most important point being how to open a swift's beak. You hold the bird in your *right* hand, Mrs. Marsault had said, and gently pull back the feathers of the top scalp, to make the beak open, and feed the bird off your left finger.

It sounded appallingly skilled to me, and I hurried upstairs thinking, 'perhaps it will be dead already', but no; it twittered on being touched, but I got no further with the food. I did not feel inclined to embark on the new technique which I was secretly terrified of, and he would not eat however much I dangled a freshly-caught fly on a paint-brush in front of his beak. I was also worried about warmth. Finally, fortified by my experience with Austin Pipper I let him sleep in my hand. He kept on twittering which kept me awake with anxiety. I felt sure he *wanted* food. Now and again I put on the bedside lamp; once or twice to my surprise he preened himself and even unexpectedly yawned, which seemed a relaxed thing to do and gave me some hope; and always he burrowed, head inwards, into my hand, into the pillow, anything, away from the light. One eye now blinked a little, and I caught a glimpse of the little black bead behind the lid.

Next morning was Sunday, 27th July, and I knew I should have to do something definite about the food.

I tried. Alas! I clearly had not got Mrs. Marsault's knack of getting the swift to open its beak by trying to pull back the top half of the skull, and I could not bring myself to persist in doing something at which I was so clumsily unsuccessful. There must be some other way. I consulted Joan Hicks' book *Their Flight Shall Continue** in which I had often found practical hints. She had had a swallow and she mentioned that when she tried to feed it, she had for the first time been faced with a firmly-closed beak. I envied her the 'first time' as I had frequently met with this dismaying situation, but never with anything so frail as a swift and requiring such difficult food. Mrs. Hicks describes how she finally got her bird to open its beak by holding it in the strong sunlight streaming through the windows, the heat causing it to gape. She then seized the opportunity to pop in a fly. This procedure continued for two days while the weather was clement, and by that time the swallow seemed to have realised that the feeding procedure was benevolent and beneficial. No more trouble. Two days! I looked out of the window, but the English weather, capricious as usual, was not going to co-operate; I felt desperate and then had an idea. I went off to find Matron and revealed my plan. I would try and open the bird's beak by having it on my knee, and using *both* hands, I would gently pull the upper and lower mandibles apart by means of the feathers, though how I was going to find anything to hold below the lower mandible I could scarcely imagine. There was only the congealed tuft. If I succeeded, then Matron ready with fly poised on paint-brush would pop it in. What I would do if it then refused to swallow—better not think of that.

We both repaired to the bathroom and I took Speedy out of his basket. I balanced him on my knee; he automatically sought to cling at an angle; feeling coldly damp, I grasped the feathers. The whole contraption seemed frailer than an eggshell and I was convinced of disaster. But no, the beak opened and Matron dexterously pushed in a fly, and, heaven be praised, it was swallowed eagerly and the little black bead glinted for a second.

In this manner Speedy consumed about thirty flies that day, also the tiniest little shreds of raw beef which he obviously enjoyed. This was an enormous relief as I blenched to think

* Published 1966. J. M. Dent & Sons Ltd.

of what one swift would need by way of flies as the mainstay of his diet. Towards evening I had a further bright idea and soaked a blue-bottle in liquid adexalin. This went down very well, and that night Speedy spent burrowed into my hairy hat in the basket, close up against the bathroom radiator.

Monday passed similarly with poor Matron frequently climbing the stairs to the bathroom.

After teaching my afternoon lesson on Monday, I set forth with my collie into a mellow evening, already a foretaste of Autumn in the air. Armed with a Colman's mustard jar and a pair of eyebrow-tweezers, flywards I was bent. I parked the car at the top of Gaudick Road, and passed under the newly-erected barrier to Paradise Woods. The barrier was bathed in sunlight, and I scanned it for blue-bottles. There were several. I muffed one or two, but caught one and dropped it into the mustard jar. I dawdled up the path. Certain plants and certain foliage seem to attract flies. I had been considered a champion fly- and mosquito-catcher of positively Graham Greenish stature in Africa. My god-daughter still recounts my exploits with awe. I trusted that my rusty expertise might regain its previous polish with practise. I made various spasmodic swipes to no effect but was elated when eventually I located and bagged eight flies on a clump of yarrow and hog-weed. As I was dropping one of these into the jar two little girls passed by and I was vaguely aware that they passed with a titter.

I strolled on and stopped opposite a conglomeration of brambles and other undergrowth. I stared hard into this rambling tangle, considering whether the beetles with yellow wing-cases on the fools' parsley, though easy to catch, would be safe nourishment for Speedy, or whether I had better confine myself to the more elusive gnats and flies unpredictably landing on and taking off from the larger bramble leaves. In the midst of this concentration, I became conscious that I was not alone. I turned abruptly to discover behind me two pink faces in the grass, also staring hard at what, I suppose, they presumed I was staring at. So now we stared at each other. At this point, my collie both bored and sensing that all was not well with the atmosphere (or 'ambience' as my students would call it), sat down and put up the prolonged howl with which he greets canned church bells on a Sunday morning. It served its purpose. I smiled; the pink faces resumed their titter, and I walked into the frayed coppice, preyed upon by prep-school 'cubs' and other rodents. It presented a very nibbled and gnawed appearance, with branches torn down, a Pepsi-Cola tin here, and an empty cigarette carton there. Leaves drifted down but not enough to camouflage the human litter beneath.

Near the pock-marked water reservoir I found a fly-fruitful patch of ivy and bramble. I heard a rustling and again felt I was being watched. Then, with a reasonable swift's-evening-meal in my jar, I hurried out of this depressing and ravaged wasteland, which had once been gracious and beautiful. I did not like its aura. As I emerged on to the open path I found myself the centre of a cloud of gnats. I waved my arms at random, and clutched at the air, thereby increasing Speedy's supper by two acceptable additions. A couple came out of the bushes and eyed me oddly, the girl even looking back over her shoulder after they had passed by.

Later that same evening Speedy seemed much stronger and suddenly ate a fly off my finger. I felt a positively lyrical uplift. He consumed roughly 50 flies, little shreds of beef, as on the day before, and a few beetle-larvae from meal-worms. I went to bed feeling greatly elated.

On Tuesday Speedy fed eagerly and drank glucose water from a teaspoon. He now climbed up the side of the basket nearest the radiator and clung (also just like a bat), to the wickerwork near the top. I kept a towel over three quarters of the basket and he always stayed where it was darkest. When you stop to think of what the nest of a swift is like, it is not surprising that Speedy should have tried to reconstruct its dark cosiness for himself.

Speedy now began to develop his personality. He would twitter every time I came into the bathroom, and scrabbled about actively in his basket, though after being fed he either went to sleep on the hairy hat at the bottom of the basket, or else climbed up and clung to the side. I also had a convalescent pigeon in the bathroom at that time, and once or twice I found Speedy crawling crab-wise towards the astonished bird. On being replaced in the basket Speedy always settled down without trouble, in fact he was the least demanding of creatures. He never ate more than three beakfuls of food at a time (i.e. two flies, one shred of beef, or 1 fly, 1 moth, 1 shred of beef, etc.). Therefore, frequency was an important factor and I had perforce to refuse all merely social engagements.

After the first three days or so, when Speedy was stronger, I decided I must do something about his eyes. I even wondered if they would ever be all right. I got the tiniest little blob of cotton wool and soaked it in Optrex slightly warmed by the addition of a drop of warm water. I held the blob to his sticky eyes, and then, very, very gently wiped a little. Speedy seemed to like this. I did very little at one go, but repeated the treatment night and morning. Gradually one eye opened completely and then the other. He did a lot of blinking at first and it was a week to ten days before the eyes were normal. I remember very well the morning when after one of these eye-baths he suddenly seemed to 'see' me. A comic expression of interest and incredulity appeared in the little beady eyes, and I had to laugh aloud. From then on he used to turn his head and take things in. Mercifully there seemed nothing wrong with his sight. The day on which he turned this corner was Saturday, 3rd August. He became very lively and also drank out of a little dish.

His appetite seemed phenomenal for so tiny a creature. I kept careful records and I give a fairly average sample of one day in Appendix II.

His first feed varied from 5.30 a.m. as on Wednesday, 31st July, to 7 a.m. (as on Thursday, 1st August) and after that it stayed steadily round about 6.30 a.m. to 7 a.m. The time of the last feeds also varied a good deal, but this depended on my use of the bathroom. If I had a bath at night, I used to leave the door open instead of putting on the light, expressly to avoid rousing Speedy, but I rarely got away with it. Persistent twitterings would issue from the basket and now he was stronger they resembled an indefatigable cricket, and I could not resist lifting him out and rewarding him with just one tit-bit—or two if required. It might be as late as 10.30 p.m. though this was exceptional, and usually there was no more feeding after half-past eight or nine.

There was a point when Speedy seemed to be excreting very little. He was rejecting flies and consuming almost only steak. This naturally worried me, but I had noticed that the nasturtiums by the West door were covered in greenfly. I scraped these off the leaves into the lid of a marmalade jar. I rolled the snippets of steak first in liquid adexalin and then in the greenfly, thus producing what my secretary referred to as 'steak garni'! It certainly did the trick. Speedy liked the adexalin oil, and the greenfly. Within 24 hours his droppings were normal both in quantity and consistency. The droppings of swallows and swifts are not liquid, but little white and black blobs which dry rather chalkily.

On Monday, 5th August, we weighed Speedy on a piece of blotting paper on the letter scales in the secretary's office. He weighed one Post Office ounce, and I wished we had weighed him when he first arrived.

I had read that Joan Hicks had given her swallow some 'daphnia'. I had not come across this before, so I went to a pet-shop and enquired. It turned out to be fish-food. I bought the smallest quantity available and introduced it to Speedy. He was not keen, but would take it if rolled in adexalin and, like the greenfly, adhering to beef snippets. I thought he really ought to have a change from beef and tried liver. This he spat out. I then tried lamb (the lean, only) and he accepted it at once with relish. I have repeatedly found that though beef, (very tender, i.e. steak!) seems the best meat on which to start a timid eater, it seems a 'heavy' kind of meat, and most birds react joyously to a change to lamb—not necessarily permanently but certainly for a short period. I usually alternate beef and lamb where I have a long convalescence.

What Speedy *did* enjoy was moths and daddy-long-legs, and one appreciated the functional width of his mouth when seeing it engulf a largish moth, wings and all. One was reminded more than ever of a frog. When one remembers that these birds catch all their food on the wing, it is not surprising that they have to be furnished in width with what the heron, for example, at the other end of the scale is furnished with in length.

On 9th August, I began to feel bothered about Speedy's flying prowess. Could he fly at all? He was now strong, and apparently with normal sight. Also he was growing in restlessness. I decided to experiment; I took him outside and threw him up into the air above the soft lawn. He spread his wings and planed down on to the grass, but without beating the air, and without any kind of steering. I repeated this two or three times, and once he came down in a clump of Michaelmas daisies, where he stayed spread-eagled, wings at full span, till I picked him up. 'The time is not yet,' I thought, but quailed at the idea of hurling him off the roof which would have given him greater height.

The next day, 10th August, a Saturday, was sunny and pleasant and again I 'exercised' Speedy in this way with two or three 'toss-ups'. The last time I thought he actually started to beat the air.

In the evening I tried again, and this time there was no mistaking Speedy's *using* his wings. He actually 'flew' a little way. I felt pleased. One of my colleagues appeared on the scene and I said, 'Would you like to see Speedy practising?' and with that I tossed him nonchalantly into the blue. He beat hard and strongly with his wings, gained height and swerved round the building. Earthbound I cantered after him in alarm, calling. He was flying bat-like before me, and the last I saw of him was as he sailed between two clumps of trees. Speedy was gone.

For the rest of the evening I searched the bushes and surroundings of the buildings in the fear that Speedy, failing to remain airborne, might have descended into them. But there was no sign. While crossing the yard I looked up to the swooping swallows, and—could it be just imagination or was there indeed wheeling among their white-breasted company, one chocolate-coloured swift? Without any intent to pun I sent the silent message—God speed!

What had originally grounded this bird?

He was young, it is true, but there was no visible damage to wing or body. I have my own theory which may be quite incorrect, and if we had known exactly *where* the swift had been found this would have helped to prove or disprove it. I have, at various times, picked up stunned birds (particularly those which swoop to catch their food on the wing) when they have flown into glass windows or similar structures. They have sometimes appeared dead, but many have revived.

The most poignant incident of this kind happened in Africa, in Uganda. I was teaching in the large new hall of the University's demonstration school which had full-length glass windows when suddenly a flock of something small flew into them in a series of moth-like thuds. I ran outside, and there, scattered on the ground, as though overtaken by some satanic holocaust, lay a shimmering collection of those enchanting little birds known by the appropriate name of 'Bronzy Mannikins'. They used to delight us by their gregarious gaiety, swinging on stalks of grass, or nimbly and apparently weightlessly climbing their slight stems. There would be a brief spell of cheerful chatter and—whoosh! —they would be gone, usually full tilt after a leader, as though playing a never-ending game of 'catch'. On this occasion they had followed him smack into the invisible glass. My class of African boys had followed me out. They were—by this time—used to my eccentricities concerning wild creatures, and what was more beginning to see and feel differently themselves. Hence there was a sincere exclamation of pity as they helped me to pick up the limp little bodies. I sat down on the step with what any uninformed passer-by would have taken to be a lapful of butterflies. There were 19 of them when I counted. I asked one of the boys to get me a mug of cold water, and while the others stood around, I administered a drop to each tiny beak. Suddenly one of the little bodies stirred and staggered drunkenly to the edge of my lap, paused and flew off, to the surprise and amusement of my pupils. Several others followed erratically. At the end of half-an-hour most of them had gone and when afternoon school was over, I had seven left lying in an African straw dish. I carried them over to the bungalow opposite the school where we lived and all but three—I think it was—revived. The last to recover took one and a half hours to regain consciousness. Presumably the three who died were the first to meet the full impact of the window. They were even smaller than Speedy, and when I first looked at his eyes I was strongly reminded of these pathetically concussed little victims.

I, therefore, concluded that Speedy had perhaps also, in his inexperienced youth, flown into a window or some other hard surface and had been pretty badly concussed. We shall never know the answer, but at least the outcome had been a happy one.

Alas, we know only too well that there are two sides to every coin. I, therefore, include the stories of my stupidities and failures because, paradoxically, they may prove more encouraging to others hesitating on the brink of action, than the stories with happy endings. Confronted with the success stories of others, I have myself acutely felt that I am the only one who ever does inexcusably idiotic things born of a lamentable combination of ignorance and a positively oafish lack of imagination. But other people's honest confessions of defeat have lessened the loneliness and have spurred me on to try again. So here is the very short story of Poppet the kestrel.

On Thursday, 8th August, the secretary told me that the Veterinary Surgeon had telephoned to say he had got something special, could I go down to the surgery to fetch it, but he would not say what it was. Luckily it was in the afternoon so I was able to go at once, bursting with curiosity. When I arrived the patient was on the table, and was a beautiful large-eyed kestrel. There appeared to be no injury, but the bird weighed less than a feather and was merely a skeleton beneath its plumage. The Veterinary Surgeon had been called on the telephone a short while before, to fetch what had sounded on the telephone like 'a sparrow'. Arrived at the address indicated he was told that the bird was under an upturned dust-bin. Inserting a hand beneath to search for the supposed 'sparrow', a kestrel had been encountered instead. The word on the 'phone leading to this misunderstanding had, of course, been 'sparrow-hawk'! I was delighted to take the bird back to be nursed, and put him in a largish cage where he collapsed on the floor. I went immediately to get some raw lamb which I cut into what I thought were reasonable pieces (about two inches by one) for a bird of prey. Please note—I had never dealt with a bird of prey before. This is not offered as an excuse but as an explanation, for here was my first mistake. The bird fell on the lamb, managed to stagger on to its feet, held the piece under one foot as I had seen a similar bird do in the Zoo, a long time ago, and after trying to tear the meat proceeded to swallow the piece whole. It did not get very far before stopping, apparently from weakness, but it recovered itself slightly and got the rest down with an effort. It did not attempt another piece. Looking back on it now I must have been demented to suppose that it was able to feed itself. I imagined that it was suffering from exhaustion (which it was) but did not realise what this *degree* of exhaustion implied. I simply thought it needed sleep and would then eat and gather strength. I took it into the bathroom for warmth and so that I could observe it. It slept, standing on the floor of the cage. I put in a few shreds of liver in case it should prefer these but it took no notice and I left it, as I told myself 'in peace'. Wise after the event I know now that this was the worst thing I could have done.

On Friday morning he looked at me with his large, beautiful eyes but did not take any interest in food. He only wanted to sleep. Even then I did not register that his only hope of survival lay in my force-feeding him. I had not realised that he was so starved that he had got beyond the point of being able to do anything about it unaided. In the evening I became alarmed and belatedly did the first sensible thing. I took the emaciated bird on to my lap and fed it some glucose water from a spoon. (I had noticed it had not even seemed thirsty, and I had not seen it drink any of the water I had put in its cage, but I did not then know that kestrels and other birds of prey practically never drink. Nevertheless it seemed grateful for the water, and I pushed down an adexalin capsule, which it swallowed docilely. I also pushed down a tiny bit of steak, put the bird back into its cage with some fresh bits of meat by its feet and left it.

How was it that I failed so miserably to understand?

Partly because it was a 'first' experience. I had never had anything so 'starved' before. Also my notions on starvation were largely based on stories of NOT allowing the starved to gorge themselves when they first met food again. I *did* know about this, and had had some experience of it. 'A little and often,' was the axiom then, I knew. But I had not encountered the stage after that where there was not enough energy left to eat. Also when I had fished an exhausted guillemot from the sea he had not eaten for three days, but had slept and rejoiced in the warmth. I had force-fed him on the third day and immediately he had started to feed himself. My basic mistake here—and heaven knows I should have known better—was to let this influence my actions with regard to the kestrel. I suspect sea-birds can, and probably do, go without food for some days because of the nature of the food. There must be times when there is a shortage of fish, and presumably they are geared to cope with these temporary famines. Moreover the kestrel had probably been for a much longer period without anything at all.

Late on Friday evening I telephoned Mrs. Marsault who advised me to try and get some more food down it, having approved the adexalin. Accordingly I visited Poppet (so-called because of his eyes). He was asleep, seemingly breathing tranquilly. It was already dark, and foolishly I could not bring myself to disturb him. That was the worst mistake I made. Had I fed him every fifteen to twenty minutes throughout the night, with glucose and milk, I cannot help feeling he might have been saved. Possibly it was too late.

On Saturday morning he was still asleep, but by this time I had woken up to the reality. I fed him another adexalin capsule, and three or four tiny bits of steak wrapped in cotton wool which had been dipped in a mixture of milk and glucose, and the tiniest drop of brandy. The wisp of cotton wool round the steak was because like owls, kestrels and other birds of prey must make pellets and need the fur or feathers (or some substitute) of their victims in order to be able to digest their food. Mrs. Marsault had reminded me of that. I now placed Poppet in a basket with a hot-water bottle under his blanket by the fire in my room. I knew now I must go all out. At that time I still thought the bird would live. I was cursing myself for my insensitive non-action, and determined now on continual small force-feeds. Half an hour later I administered another two snippets of steak, obediently swallowed but without any sign of relish or pleasure. I also gave a quarter of a tablet of vitamin B. I noticed the bird's breathing was quick and began to worry as to the actual seriousness of its condition. I returned in half-an-hour after telephoning the Veterinary Surgeon to report on the bird and to tell him what I was doing. Poppet was dead.

I was shocked beyond measure. There was a dreadful emptiness. Knowing that I myself certainly seemed to be the sole cause of this cessation of life, I was too distressed to try to analyse my deficiencies at this point. The Veterinary Surgeon already overburdened with the living, most generously consented to do a post-mortem. It revealed what had already been diagnosed that there was no visible cause for death other than starvation and exhaustion.

I thought long and frequently about this. It is salutary to become aware of one's preconceived ideas. I had approached the kestrel, in its dire need with far too many ready-made notions. First of these was a largely unconscious idea that birds of prey were 'tough'. They may be, but nevertheless subject to the same vulnerabilities common to all organic life, amongst which the absence of food must take priority. Secondly, I have a purely personal inclination to feel that sleep and 'to-be-left-in-peace' is usually more important than food. It often is, *but* naturally not always, and I am sure that the kestrel was a spectacular example of where this approach was so wide of the mark as to prove fatal. And then, in some way, I had been far too confident. This is always disastrous. I tend to think if there is no fearsome injury the chances of the patient's recovery are infinitely greater. There are no sound grounds for such a supposition. My general feeling had been 'This bird is underfed (a euphemism) and worn out. We'll give him peace, warmth and food, and all will be well.' A far too facile conclusion. I ought to have said to myself, 'This bird is so weak, owing to starvation and exhaustion that it is at death's door, and only constant and unremitting attention, plus force-feeding can even give it the slimmest hope of recovery.' I had learnt an unforgettable lesson but the cost—to me, at least—was too high. I shall never forget the extreme *gentleness*, almost the *courtesy*, of this lovely bird, the cobweb softness of its autumn bracken-coloured plumage, and the haunting resignation in its eyes.

CHAPTER SIX

Mossy Moussec–Orphan of the Storm

Outside in the Park the trees roared and the pale blue lightning sent my collie cowering against my bed. Yet it was May, the month of baby birds. Storms automatically direct my thoughts to birds. The crashing sea would bring in the oiled sea-birds, helpless, floundering victims of man's greed; and inland—who could tell? Branches cracked and leaves scampered over the grass as though they were alive. On Tuesday, 13th May, Miss Raymonde-Hawkins of the Raystede Animal Rescue Centre telephoned to say she would be bringing me a baby owl found in the hospital grounds at Handcross. He duly arrived in a Raystede 'Pussy-pack'. Indeed he was scarcely distinguishable from some exaggeratedly fluffy kitten, or ball of angora wool.

I selected an oval basket with a handle. It had been especially made for me as a farewell present by the African girls in a junior school in Uganda. It was ideal. In went the hot-water bottle wrapped in a vest, and over the handle a towel. Into this snug retreat I tipped the new arrival. He snuggled up to the hot-water bottle and revealing two dark glass-button eyes voiced a reminder that the best hotels do not neglect the menu. It was after seven in the evening, but I keep some lean lamb in the frig for Binkie, the crippled blackbird. I cut a little into small portions (about the size of a finger-nail), rapidly combed some fur out of my astonished collie, snipped it up with scissors, and having soused the lamb in minced fur and allowed it to warm up to room temperature, proffered it on the end of eye-brow tweezers. It met with unqualified approval.

As I gazed at him (and he at me) I realised vividly why Dorothy Yglesias had called her first baby owl the 'Abominable Snowman'. Nothing could have been more appropriate; there was something snowy, frothy about his fluff, that inevitably recalled the frostiness of winter moss. His 'fizziness' evoked my own preference for rather naïvely fizzy drinks, and so his name was born. I have never been able to afford champagne, and have always happily made do on special occasions with Moussec, not wholly unclouded with a guilt feeling that even this was unjustified self-indulgence.

All my life I had longed for a baby owl. As a child I had found one bloated with one of those transparent air-sacs, like some huge water-blister. I had not dared to prick it and the owl had died. Now here, as far as one could tell, was a healthy fledgeling, orphan of the storm, and for me a dream fulfilled.

But what did I know about rearing owls? Once more I was facing a first experience with the member of a new species and all its attendant doubts and gropings. One is working in the dark, conscious only of one's ignorance and dreading its possibly fatal results. I went to bed and woke up at intervals to feed the ever-ready beak.

The first day passed off without incident. Mossy Moussec slept, but came lurching to the opening in the towel whenever he became aware of food. That night I decided to pick him up. I had, so far not handled him. When I had him in my hands I was startled to find his abdomen round and hard as a cricket ball. Immediately ghastly fantasies crowded upon me. True he had discreetly excreted one or two miniature whipped cream walnuts, resembling those sold singly in combined tobacconist-sweet shops, and in his case cream-coloured and decorated with a chain of what looked like high-class caviar. Was that all there should be? It was already 10.30 p.m. and I dared not telephone Mrs. Marsault for advice. There was the night to be got through and suppose Moussec was stuck and required relieving? He seemed more restless. Finally I painted the vent with warm salad oil, and also cautiously administered about a small teaspoonful of slightly warmed salad oil orally. Moussec took this in his stride but a little whimperingly and shortly after excreted an evil-smelling splodge of black excretion. 'Now he's got diarrhoea,' I thought desperately. Finally dawn came with

Moussec asleep and me awake.

At a reasonable hour I telephoned Mrs. Marsault. Her understanding, competent, and reassuring voice did wonders. She pointed out that owls' stomachs appeared below the breast-bone and said she too had had a baby owl with the cricket-ball abdomen and had massaged it and applied some sort of oil. (Vegetable oil, of course, *not* mineral oil such as liquid paraffin.) I put down the receiver considerably relieved, and went to the basket. Moussec was asleep, his head flat out beside the hot-water bottle, exactly like a baby. Perhaps it was going to be all right after all.

I have since learnt that there was, in fact, nothing abnormal about poor Moussec's stomach, and after my first unjustified alarm all went smoothly. A week went by, and when I celebrated the date of his arrival I heaved a sigh of relief that we had got so far. At this stage Mossy Moussec ate slivers of lamb's liver and bits of lean lamb rolled either in minced dog fur or in small, fluffy pigeon's feathers. Moussec seemed to be flourishing but when no pellet appeared I again found myself asking questions I could not answer. At what age and stage does a fledgeling owl begin to cast pellets? And is it possible for an owl to form pellets without bone? In its natural state it would be getting mice and baby birds.

I sent out urgent messages to friends with cats, to ask them to try and salvage a few mice, making sure that these could not possibly have been poisoned. Various indignant cats were deprived of their prey but the supply was thin and chancy. The first mouse I got, I forced myself to chop into three. Moussec devoured the head in the morning, the middle in the afternoon and at 5 p.m. the mouse's tail was realistically wriggling at the end of his beak. Clearly I had to find suitable substitutes. The Veterinary Surgeon, who was deeply interested in Moussec's development, suggested rabbit ribs. I bought half a New Zealand rabbit, pounded the ribs and flesh into a pulp with a hammer and fed it to Moussec who seemed pleased. He produced his first somewhat squashy pellet after five days and thereafter a pellet appeared at approximately three- or five-day intervals.

Accidentally I caught sight of a notice in a shop in Seaside which said, 'chicken giblets 1s. 6d. a pound'. Moussec greatly appreciated these and the pulped neck added to his intake of bone. I never fed him more than an inch of this pulp at a time.

Then there was the question of water. Ordinary small fledgelings are grateful for one or two drops of water taken from a small camel-hair brush and later from a small teaspoon. I tried a few drops in a teaspoon with Moussec. (One must be careful with this, or else too much water goes down and the bird chokes just as a baby would.) As Moussec registered what was happening an interested look dawned in his eyes which changed to obvious pleasure. Once he had swallowed he expressed his satisfaction by 'tasting' with loud and uninhibited smacking noises; just as a human being 'smacks his lips' so Moussec was 'smacking his beak'. You could see his tongue waggling. On Monday, 19th May, six days after his arrival, he drank by himself out of a Turkish coffee cup held out to him. He never drank a great deal, but there was no mistaking his enjoyment.

In the fifth week of his stay he suddenly tried to bath in the coffee cup! He dipped his head and went through all the movements of throwing water over his back. I hastily fetched my salad bowl and he had his first rather incompetent bath. His plus-fours clung to his feathered legs but he did not succeed in bathing higher up. He seemed complacent about his performance and I vowed to myself that I would have him photographed in his bath. Alas, he left before I could arrange it.

Soon after his arrival Moussec started his 'nibbling'. First of all he nibbled the clean tissues I put at the bottom of the basket (alongside the wrapped hot-water bottle). He soon had these in shreds. I had a feeling he was trying to get extra 'roughage' to aid his digestive processes but I never saw him actually swallowing the tissue. It appeared to give him some sort of satisfaction, however, but then he nibbled round the edge of his basket. It was made of plaited banana leaves. I tried to visualise his natural habitat and what he would be nibbling there. Finally I fetched a piece of soggy, rotten branch, containing a few small insects, the kind which Jack Devon, the jackdaw, had so much enjoyed—and at once Moussec diverted his nibbling to the wood. He *did* actually eat bits of soft wood, and from then on it was necessary to furnish him with rotten wood daily. At a later stage he used to hold pieces in his foot while he nibbled and ate, rather like a child with a toffee-apple. Sometimes he just tore the wood into pieces. He ate wood-lice, but I did not think that the insects in the wood (they were so very small and not many) constituted his primary interest. He was just as happy with barren bits. Then I noticed him nibbling and eating bits of the beech-leaves I had in a vase of flowers. Experimentally, I got a bunch of chickweed as the small birds like it so much. Moussec loved it. He was, of course, enjoying a full diet of 'fake mice'. His favourite diet now was chicken livers and hearts, wrapped (as already stated) in pigeon's fluffy feathers or in finely chopped dog fur or sheep's wool (from a student's discarded sheepskin hat)! He also relished the kidney from the steak and kidney sold ready mixed in butchers' shops. He preferred it 'au naturel' unwrapped and did not like the steak on which he turned an insulted eye. Moussec loved brain, also unwrapped. The texture of what he enjoyed is significant. He liked all 'floppy meat' reminiscent of the limpness of recently killed things. He was by no means a greedy eater and in the course of twenty-four hours his intake was, I suppose, roughly the equivalent of four mice. After his very early days he would not touch lamb. So my dog had that. Indeed, he was both delighted and perplexed by this halcyon period during which he lived on steak, best rabbit and Moussec's overflow of chicken giblets. After Moussec's departure he greeted his return to the mundane pet's mince or breast of lamb with questioning looks and sighs of resignation.

Moussec lived with me in my room and was never confined. During his early residence in the basket, it was placed on a chair at a convenient feeding level. Gradually he emerged and perched for short periods first on the edge of the basket, then on its handle and from there he wing-hopped on to the arm and back of the couch beside the chair. Once he began to fly and to shed some of his baby-fluff, he used to roost either on the wooden curtain-rod or on the top of the door which always stands open as it merely leads to my small entrance landing.

I have three windows in my room and at least one of these is always open at the top. Moussec used to sit on the ledge half-way up the window and gaze concentratedly through the pane. When he had had enough he retired to one of his usual roosts.

Once over babyhood he established the rhythm of his routine. He slept during the day, though he would eat a little if I held it out to him about lunch-time. He began to get lively around 6.30 p.m. and then he would pounce fiercely on the sheep-skin rug, fix the dog with unwinking eye and occasionally ride on his back. Finally he would perch on the back of my armchair and nibble my ear or my hair.

One night, after a lecture-demonstration, I had the lecturer, who is a good friend of the College, to supper in my room. He is an admirable lecturer and was enthusing about our next venture, when he suddenly leant forward and said with a dazed stare 'Good God! That's an owl!' Moussec had taken up his usual statuesque stance on the back of my chair.

Moussec would have supper, or, presumably, his breakfast, at about 7 p.m. He ate again before I went to bed, and I used to leave him sitting on a special portable perch I'd had constructed and which I used to put by the window for him. At 12.30 a.m., at 2.30 a.m., and at 4.30 a.m., he would come to the chair near my bed and wake me by calling. I had his food ready in the kitchen and after he had had his feed I went to sleep again. In the morning when I made myself a cup of tea at 6.30 a.m., he would sometimes lie on my shoulder and go to sleep. When I got up I would hoist him to his perch on top of the door, and after, perhaps, another snack, he would settle down for his snooze through the day.

A word about this 'lying down'. I had grown accustomed to seeing Moussec lying down in his characteristic baby way in his basket, but the first time I ever saw him recumbent after he became active outside his basket I was completely unprepared and sure he had met with an accident.

He appeared as a collapsed bundle of feathers on top of the monkey's cage situated on the table in front of the built-in mirror in my room. Moussec had previously stared into the mirror and when I saw this fluffy heap of owl I was certain he had flown at the mirror and fallen concussed on the top of the cage. I was quite wrong. Subsequently when Moussec 'lay down' for a quiet siesta in various places, including my pillow and shoulder I observed very clearly the same complete abandonment to sleep. I longed to get a photograph of this but owls do not lie down to order and I never managed to record this particular picture of repose.

Moussec was extremely fastidious concerning personal cleanliness. He was always spotless and had a lovely heathery smell. This fastidiousness would seem to be a characteristic, interestingly enough and, according to human concepts, perhaps rather paradoxically, of birds of prey. Later when Tiger Tim, the kestrel, shared my room, he exhibited the same symptoms. Moussec paid great attention to pedicure. He would delicately and carefully go round the claws of each foot, after which operation he would spread one out in front of him and gaze at it with the—to coin an adjective—manicurial absorption frequently assumed by female shop assistants when bent on ignoring their customers.

If at any time Moussec felt threatened or annoyed, as when some unforeseen situation arose such as the monkey approaching him while out for his daily exercise, he would spread his wings and sharply snap his beak. This beak-snapping and general pluffing-out of feathers and wings was clearly meant to warn off intruders.

At the end of six weeks to two months Moussec grew more restless at night and spent longer periods staring out of the window. He now preferred me to put his food down and he would pounce on it and tear it with the help of his foot.

Then one evening when I had two friends in my room, he flew to the open window and perched half in and half out. After about an hour he turned round, flew back into the room and for the first time in his life sat in the middle of the dog's plate and started to stuff down the dog's supper, rice and all. 'He's getting ready for the great adventure,' said one of my friends. Early next morning I felt his wing brush my cheek.

I did not immediately rouse myself and when I did so about twenty minutes later, the room was empty and he was gone.

At 6 a.m. I discovered Moussec asleep on top of the column by the South door. I stood below and called. He opened one eye and immediately shut it again. I called again and he flew into the neighbouring ilex, which caused the usual chattering consternation among the small birds. He ignored them. Two jackdaws approached with obviously aggressive intentions but to my relief he sent them packing with great efficiency. I visited the ilex every half an hour but at 10.30 a.m. Moussec had disappeared. I saw him later in the day in the wood round the margin of our Park, and again the next day. He would not come to me but flew out of one tree and into another. After that I lost sight of him. We all missed him and I had heard terrible stories about the difficulty of releasing hand-reared owls. I placed my hopes in the fact that Moussec had never been in a cage, and had always had free access to the open. I hoped, therefore, that his evolution in this respect had resembled to some extent what would have been his normal development in a natural environment.

Just over a fortnight later on a Sunday in July, we had an appalling storm. A Force 9 gale was registered which rocked the caravans at Pevensey Bay. I lay awake and thought of Moussec. The following afternoon the Bursar telephoned my office and said 'Have you got your owl out in the Park? Because there's an owl lolloping around under the kitchen window.' I rushed into the Park. There was Moussec, looking dazed and battered in the clumps of Herb Robert below the kitchen window. I called 'Moussec' and ran towards him. He lifted his head and uttered pitiful whimpers. I gathered him up, hurried indoors, filled a hot-water bottle and put him back where he started life with me—in his basket with the towel over it. He promptly went to sleep while I dashed into the town for a pound of chicken giblets. On my return he ate ravenously. For the first twenty-four to thirty-six hours he slept and woke up only to eat. Then he returned to all his old habits and usual routine.

He had lost a lot more of his fluffy feathers and his ears showed. On Thursday he became restless once more and on

Friday evening he ate a large supper. At 9.45 p.m. on my return from a student picnic, he ate two pieces of kidney, but looking round alertly. During this time I had kept the window open at the top only, and the gap measured about five inches. I went into the kitchen to fetch something and on re-entering my room, saw that Moussec had squeezed into the gap of the window from which he had made his previous exit. I said rather primly, 'Moussec, you know what happened last time. Don't you think you had better stay a bit longer?' For answer he launched himself as well as he could through the restricted space and flew into the clump of beeches opposite my window.

That is really the documentary end of Moussec's story, but I would like to report that he landed on my window-sill the night after his departure and answered my call for several nights after that. And four evenings ago (23rd July), one of the men from the estate who occasionally patrols the Park and is well-acquainted with its wild life, very kindly called to tell me he had seen Moussec, apparently in good trim, by the little summerhouse in the wood. He knew it was my owl, as it was tamer than the usual ones and was alone, whereas, he said, the established owl inhabitants were two elderly couples normally seen together.

I had learnt a great deal. In addition to many other things I had learnt that apart from casting pellets—not necessarily regularly, but depending on the intake of roughage—the droppings of an owl are of two kinds; the black splodges and the cream-coloured. After Moussec ceased to be a nestling his creamy droppings lost their cream-cheese consistency and became loose.

I had learnt that a convenient way of supplying bone was by means of pulped rabbit ribs and chicken necks, and that Moussec at least appeared to require wood and some green stuff to nibble as part of a healthy diet.

Above all, due to my fortunate position in the middle of ancient and wooded grounds, it had been possible to return Moussec to his natural environment.

Now all that remained was to wish him good hunting and domestic happiness.

CHAPTER SEVEN

The Pigeon's Lot

'Are we going to have pigeon-turds on toast again?' remarked my god-daughter brightly, looking round my kitchen where I was preparing a delicious grilled rainbow trout à la mayonnaise. Her observation had—it is true—its foundation in fact, as on her previous visit she had, alas, when about to place some slices of bread under the grill, found unmistakable clues signalling 'pigeons'. This was because I had collected one of the many exhausted racing pigeons which, battered by the storms of the Channel, arrive on the coast, cold, hungry, near the end of their tether, and then collapse on the Downs. I had noticed this one, trying to pick up the weed-seeds which fall from the verge on to the asphalt at the side of the road. Its movements had betokened a very weary pigeon indeed. I got out of the car, but it still had strength to haul itself into the air only to flop down a few yards further on. I did not wish to exhaust it further to no purpose, but I feared the traffic. Sure enough, on my return down the same road half an hour later, there it was lying almost where I had left it. It was still alive and not badly injured. Luckily for the pigeon its tail had been run over and wrenched off, probably saving its life.

I took it with me, and as with all similar patients put it in the wooden fruit-bowl on the draining-board by the kitchen-window. I put a little dish of mixed corn, and also a drink of water, by the bowl. The pigeon blinked in a semi-dazed condition but soon registered the food and drink and set to. To help her over the shock, I placed a hot-water bottle leaning over the bowl against the wall. This was the start of 'turds on toast'! This unassuming little patient was always beautifully behaved, quiet and contented, never restless, but when she felt better and exercised her wings a little, she would fly on to the gas-stove and back to the draining-board. On the gas-stove, however, she discovered that kettles which had just been boiled were warm, and one chilly evening, after having enjoyed a 'cuppa', I came into the kitchen to find pigeon (she never had a name) wistfully snuggled up against the kettle.

This led to the occasional penny on the toast-rack beneath!

In those days I was very green about racing pigeons, so conscientiously I traced the owner via the number on the ring round its leg, and received a very pleasant reply to my letter. Its owner lived in Somerset, and in due course, some weeks later, I went up to Victoria Station, and placed the pigeon, travelling in my cat-basket, on the passenger train, and as arranged, sent a telegram announcing the time of the pigeon's arrival at its destination. It was collected, and with the return of my basket I had an appreciative note to say the pigeon was in fine condition and soon a new tail would replace the old, qualifying it once more to race. This gave me to think.

One of Tom Lehrer's macabre lyrics 'Poisoning Pigeons in the Park', like the rest of his vitriolic satire is accurately observed and reflects the official—and largely also, the popular—attitude.

'Pigeons are vermin; there are too many of them and they are destructive,' otherwise sentimentally* inclined acquaintances are wont to remark. Well, if that is an acceptable definition of vermin, then human beings hold first-class qualifications for the title; there are far too many of them too, and their destructiveness is unparallelled.

Poison, enteritis and injuries mostly due to cars combined with starvation, are the three commonest causes of pigeon distress in my experience. In addition there are the birds without actual injury, usually racing pigeons, suffering from exhaustion and starvation.

Against poison, mostly from the effects of poison sprays and seed dressings, there is little or nothing to be done; its most

* I use the word with due consideration. People find it easy to be sentimental about animals and birds and in my experience sentimentality is most frequently linked with cruelty.

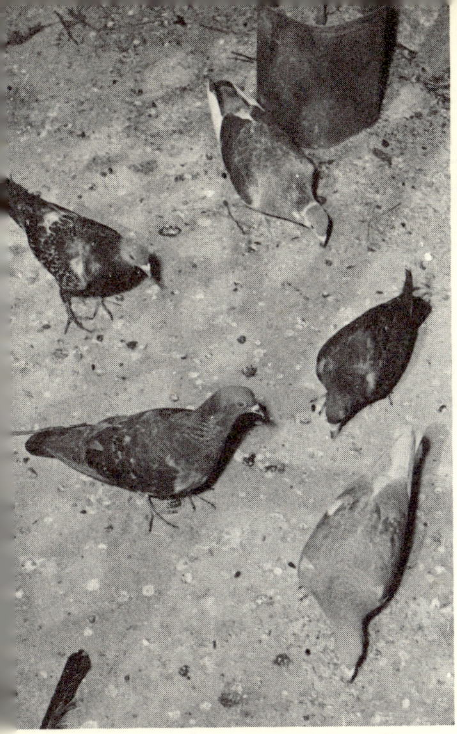

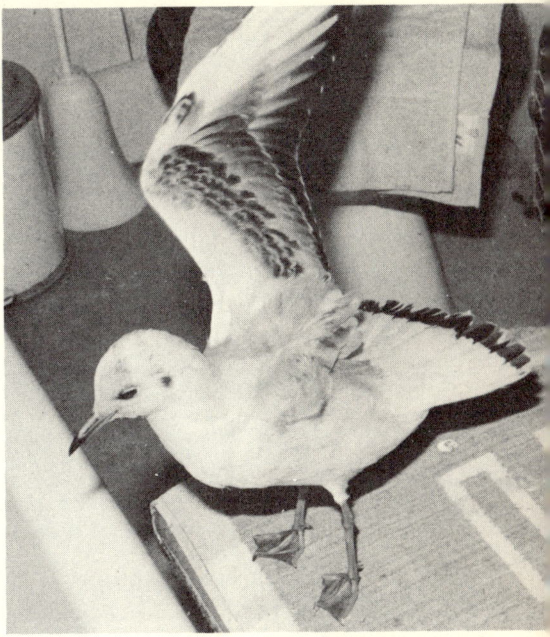

(Left). Pattern of pigeons. (Right). Nelson (bathroom patient). Small black-headed gull with amputated left wing. This wing was completely gangrened.

(Left). Guillemot, just before being de-oiled. Note the feet. This bird made a good recovery. (Right). The same guillemot the day after being de-oiled, having had several good meals!

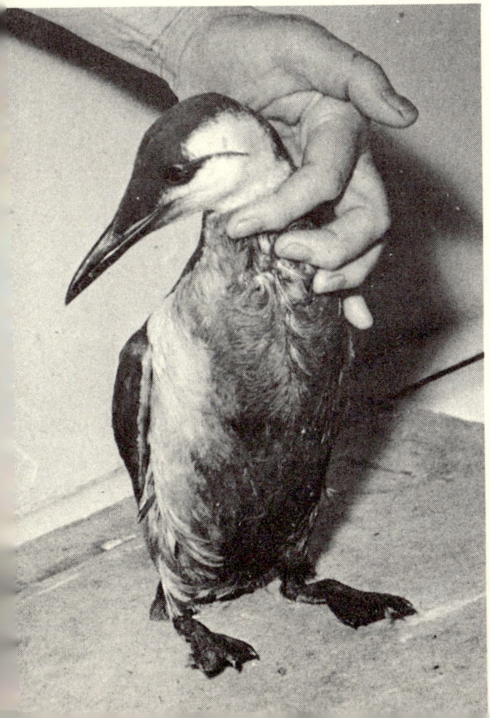

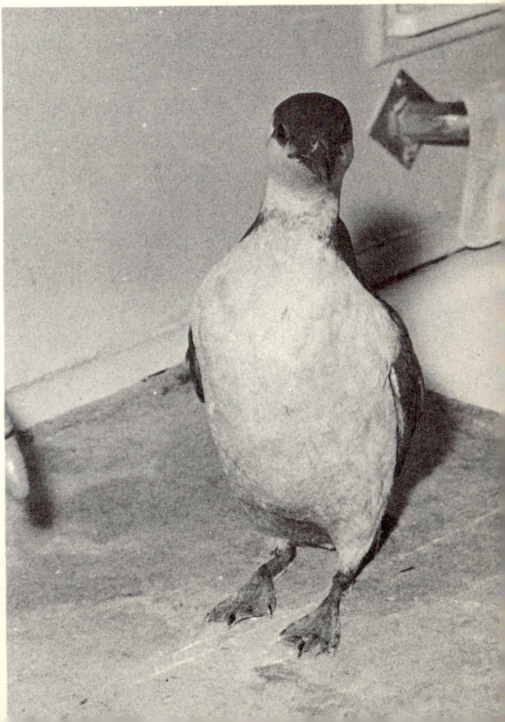

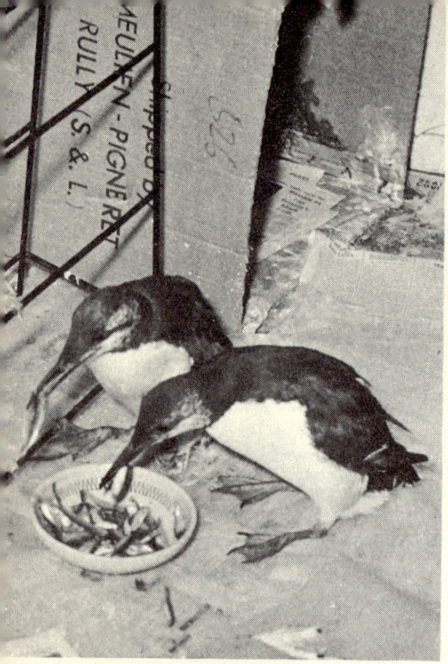

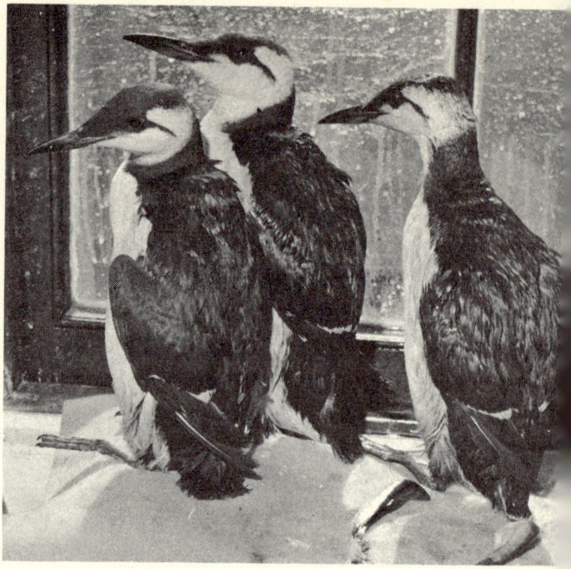

(Above, Left). Bathroom patients. Two guillemots (de-oiled) eating. (Above, Right). Mr. Kwak (nearest window) anticipating more fun. Janni (next to Mr. Kwak) thoughtful and grave. The Mini-guillie (behind on right) looking towards 'the boys'.

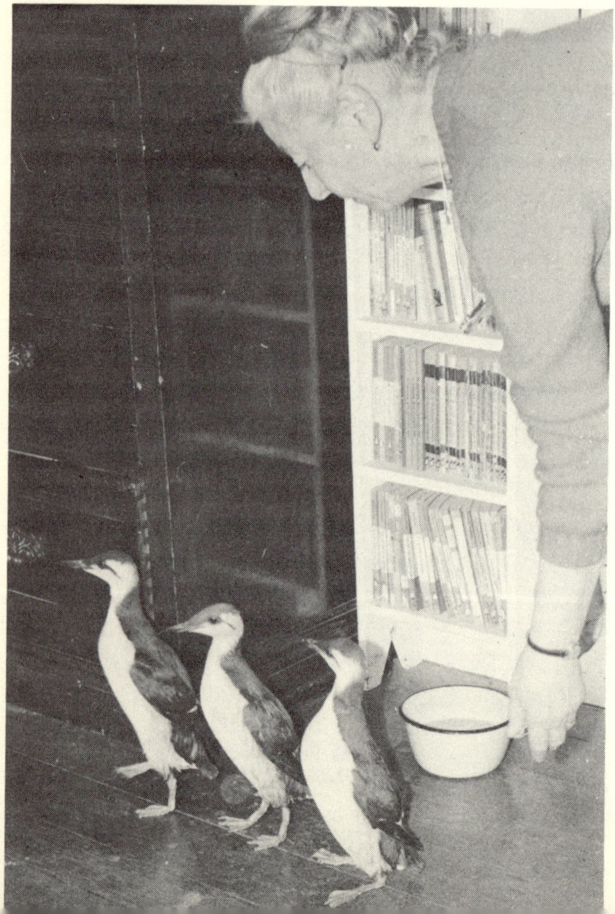

Janni, the Mini-guillie and Mr. Kwak, in good marching order, on their way to the window-seat.

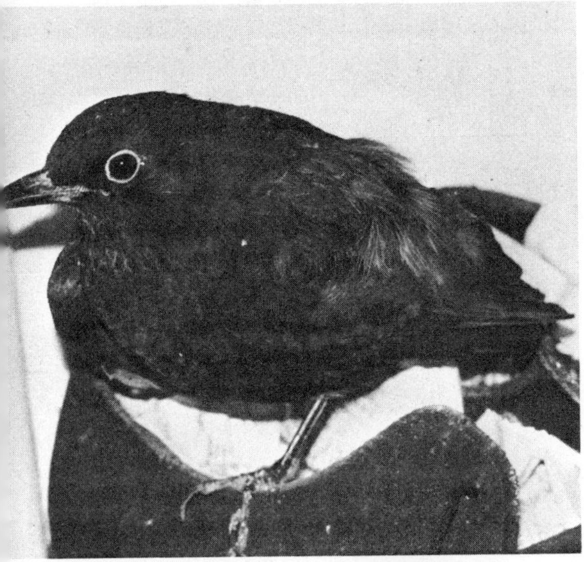

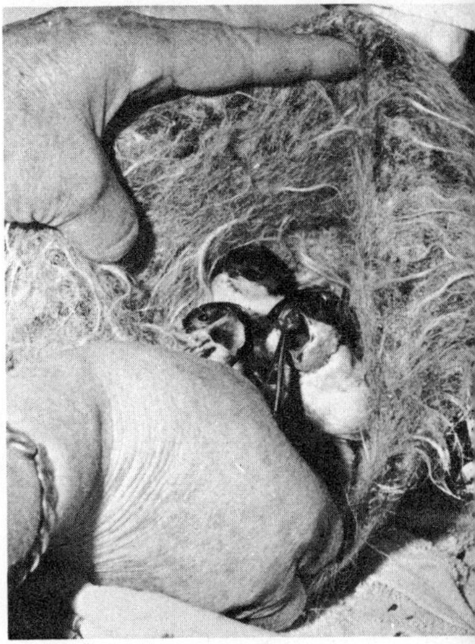

(Above). Binkie the gallant, roosting on my shoe.

(Above, Right). Minet, Manet and Monet being fed inside their 'hairy hat' nest.

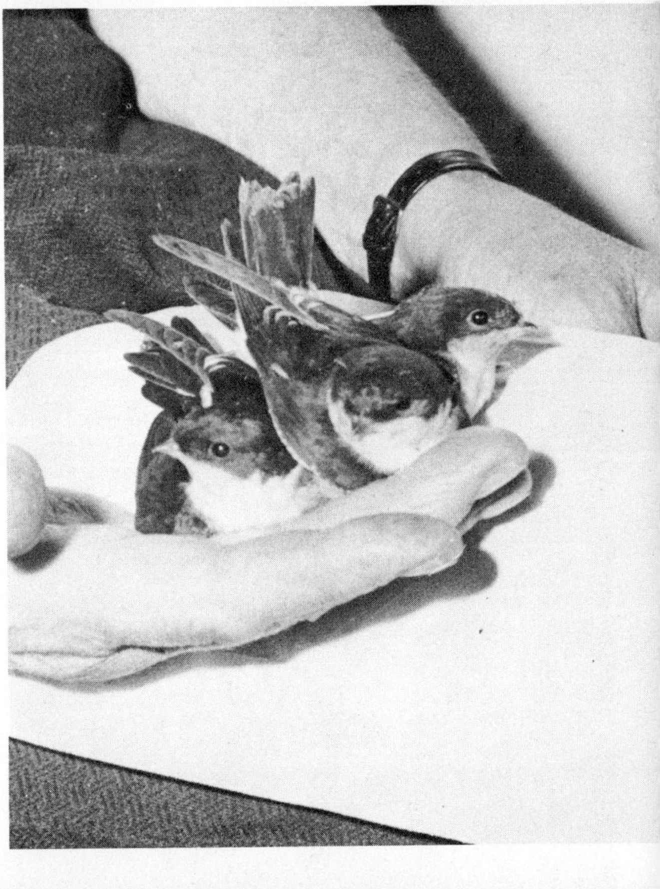

(Right). A nestful of house-martins; Minet, Manet and Monet again.

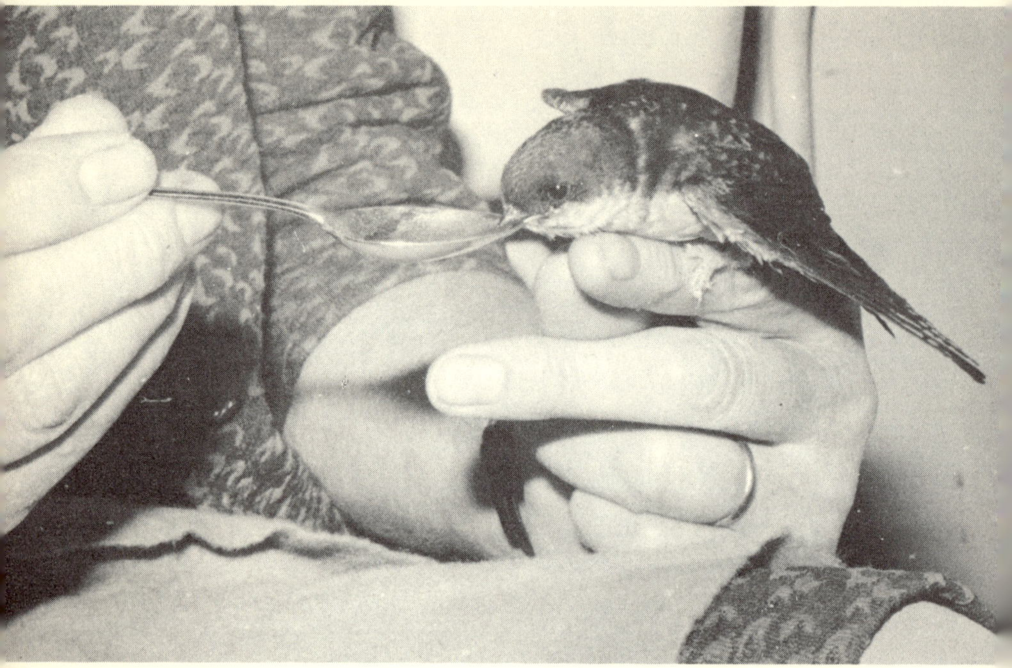

House-martin drinking from small teaspoon.

Cuckoo eating mealworm.

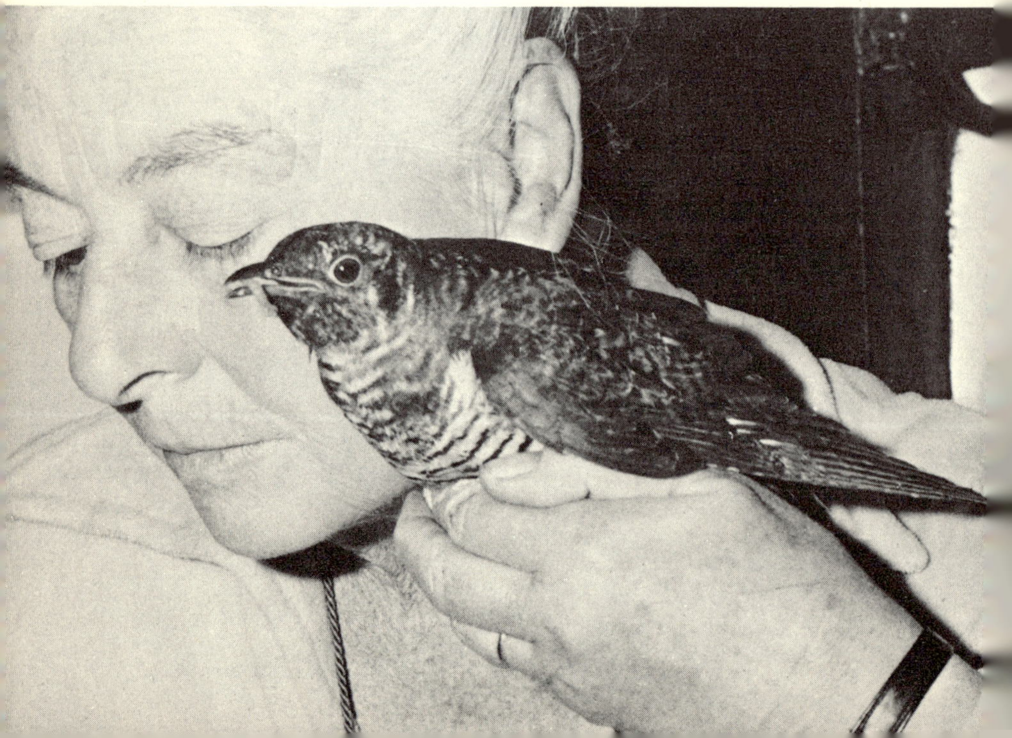

recognisable feature is the viridian green colour of the bird's droppings. One can only keep the bird warm and quiet, in semi-darkness, let it drink, and at least the helpless vulnerability of its condition will no longer add the agony of terror to its physical pain. By the time one finds such birds helpless they rarely live for longer than another twenty-four hours, generally only for a few hours, and frequently die writhing in convulsions.

Enteritis is usually a result of some kind of poisoning also, but it can be due to other causes, such as dirt or food which is polluted but not to the degree which causes death. In that case the first thing I do is to force-feed a capsule of the intestinal antiseptic, Dianimol (a little diluted), and keep the pigeon under constant observation. This means the patient is either in my kitchen or in the bathroom, according to its mobility. If too sick to be mobile, then it has the fruit-bowl on the draining-board in the kitchen; if slightly mobile then it goes into the bathroom where it can walk about if it wants to. Even if the patient is a bathroom patient, it is immediately placed in a basket with a hot-water bottle wrapped in something soft. Sometimes, if not too sick, the birds are ready to eat and drink straight away; if not, this is usually a sinister sign with pigeons who seem remarkably tough and will eat even just after a fracture has been splinted or strapped. They eat with such an expression of shy delight in the eye, and look at one so gratefully, that they would disarm all but those beyond the pale of human mercy. I am profoundly touched by the commonest of common pigeons on these occasions.

Indeed were the pigeon not 'common' what panegyrics would be composed in its honour. Who but the most leathern-hearted denier of life can fail to find delight in their shimmering rainbow colours, the classical simplicity of form, magnificently caught by Picasso (in his painting, 'Girl with a Pigeon'), the carnelian eyes, the prim little coraline feet with the ebony toe-nails, delicate as the design of veins in an ivy leaf, the sturdy grace of gesture and movement on the ground—the strong wheeling flight patterned against the lucid or cloudy sky, and the low, lovable cooing.

The first of my pigeons to become a permanent lodger was Bertie.

I was attending a weekend Teachers' Course at Exeter, and knowing that Mrs. Marsault scarcely knew where to turn, having been inundated with *Torrey Canyon* casualties, I had offered to relieve her of at least one straightforward 'case', should she feel inclined to trust me. I had imagined, heaven knows why, it would be a sea-bird. I had promised to ring her up from Exeter. Accordingly, having issued from a lecture which had left me distinctly limp, I was pleased to hear Mrs. Marsault's crisp and astringent tones on the telephone.

'Would you take an amputated crow?'

'A what?'

'An amputated crow?'

'An amputated crow?' I was trying to rearrange my images.

'Yes, well, I'm not quite sure yet. I may have to take out another little bit of bone. In that case I'd better hang on to her and you could have an amputated pigeon.'

I fixed a time to visit Mrs. Marsault to view the amputation cases during our 'free' afternoon. The amputated crow turned out to be in need of further surgical attention. I was sneakingly relieved at this for 'Charlotte', as she had been named, glowered at me with Bronte-esque grimness, whereas the one-legged pigeon, unnamed as yet, exhibited signs of a more extroverted nature. It was decided I should call in to fetch him on my way back to Eastbourne. The next day after a welcome coffee in the kitchen, Mrs. Marsault tenderly and clearly reluctantly, placed the pigeon in my cat-basket, with the words, 'I have *never* let *anyone* have any of my birds before.' I was acutely aware of both the honour and the responsibility, and swore to myself that I would never, never face Mrs. Marsault again, should anything go wrong.

I had decided to call the pigeon 'Bertie'. He looked 'Bertie' to me. He had been captured by children in a shelter and they had 'played at racing pigeons' with him. This meant they had 'ringed' him, with an elastic band, so tightly that he got gangrene. The lower half of his leg had dropped off (Mrs. Marsault had preserved it in a matchbox) and had he not had the timely good fortune to receive expert attention and sustained nursing, he would have suffered an inexcusably lingering death.

Bertie, therefore, was now merely in need of 'convalescent home' care.

He started off indoors, with day and night personal service so that we could get to know each other. Mrs. Marsault had given me a little sponge rubber pad for his 'stump' should this be required. However, Bertie flourished, ate well and showed no discomfort, other than occasionally missing his footing by relying on a bit of leg that wasn't there. As the weather grew warmer I decided to put him in the small stable which served as a semi-open-air 'aviary'. It already had a roughly constructed 'pigeon-cote' attached to the wall, high up under the roof. I had put a large branch of a tree just underneath, and various smaller birds had completed successful convalescent periods in this halfway house to freedom.

Bertie established himself, and became its pampered, permanent resident. From time to time he shared his spacious apartment with others, and whenever he became unnecessarily assertive, Matron would always defend him—'After all; he *was* the first.'

Though not unamiable—he would coo at Matron and myself —he retained a surly reserve towards strangers, particularly children, for which, after his experiences, he could hardly be blamed.

I sent regular bulletins on his progress to Mrs. Marsault. After a year I thought it would be agreeable for Bertie, who was now exceedingly handsome, to extend his activities, by opening the top half of the inner stable door. I had had an inner door made of wire netting, so that when the outer door was open, there was plenty of light and air as well as security. I naturally took no steps without consulting Mrs. Marsault. She agreed that Bertie, now wholly adjusted to his physical handicap, would probably appreciate greater freedom. The next fine day, not without a certain degree of trepidation, I opened the top half of the inner door and then hid to watch. Bertie rolled a marmalade eye at the unfamiliar gap, but evinced no further interest. Work pressed, so I left him. Later on, however, there he was making a Long John Silver tour of the courtyard. Apparently he approved for thenceforth he came out daily, but returned to his pigeon-cote lodge at night. Then I shut the door to make sure he was safe.

In due course he returned with a nervous girl-friend, petite and pretty, who gave the impression that she had been led astray before and no amount of cooing cajolery on the part of Bertie would persuade her to enter the stable. She disappeared, and Bertie next brought along a buxom pigeon-lass whose homely looks promised more likely domestic bliss. And indeed, she inspected the stable and settled into the pigeon-cote; Bertie, rather incompetently, fussed around with twigs, but Flossie as we called her, was clearly the one to wear the trousers and the dominant nest-builder. Finally two eggs were laid and we awaited events.

The events, however, failed to take place. One day we found broken egg-shells and Bertie was left a grass widower. He sulked around for a bit, and then stayed out for the odd night or two. He always returned as he was very fond of peanuts, and I doubted whether he would take up residence elsewhere. I was wrong, or else some unforeseen fate overcame him. He did not return, and we missed him greatly. I told Mrs. Marsault, who was inclined to take the view that he had met with disaster. I am not altogether sure about this for we have elderly neighbours who live in great seclusion and I am told their great joy is to feed numbers of wild birds, amongst whom are various kinds of pigeons and doves. It is possible that Bertie had set up house somewhere in the vicinity, though admittedly it is equally if not more likely that he has been shot by those trigger-happy disposers of birds in general and pigeons in particular.

This raises the question, to free or not to free one's pigeons. Personally I feel they should be given their independence, even though this involves hazards. I could have kept Bertie locked up in the stable. There was plenty of room. He was warm and well-fed. On the other hand, he gazed out on the activity of the courtyard, the sunshine, other pigeons and natural food. He need never have wandered had he not felt so inclined. Rightly or wrongly, I have continued to give my recovered pigeons free choice to come or go.

During the latter part of Bertie's sojourn, other pigeons and doves kept coming and going. They were a mixed lot, so I will select a few 'cases' from my records in order to give a roughly representative cross-section.

SQUEAKER

When the Veterinary Surgeon first rang me up to say diffidently and negatively, 'You wouldn't take a pigeon, would you?' I laughed and said, 'Of course I would. What's wrong with it?' 'Generally bashed about,' came the quietly terse reply, and I asked no more. There rose before me the vision of yet another 'bashed about' pigeon which Mrs. Marsault had personally rescued from its tormentors. She had prized a pebble out of its head and had saved its life. I had seen the pebble which had been fired by a catapult.

I went down to the surgery and fetched a very frightened, dirty and not wholly grown-up bird. It still 'bleeped' like a squab though it was self-feeding. Everyone in the surgery smilingly remarked on the piercing nature of its bleeps, and these continued as I carried the basket along the pavement to the car.

Inevitably the bird was christened 'Squeaker'. He started as a bathroom patient, and redoubled his bleeps in excitement over his food (Bertie had never been content with less than the best!) coupled with his obvious, touchingly increasing belief in a new-found security. After a period of adjustment Squeaker was duly decanted into the stable aviary. He bathed copiously which resulted in gleaming, iridescent plumage.

'Where's that dreary-looking bird you had?' the odd visitor would remark, and when proudly I pointed out the renewed Squeaker, they would exclaim, 'No! Are you sure it's the same one? How do you know?'

After his first moult Squeaker emerged gorgeously and positively an unmistakable 'he'. He is still with me and boss of the stable 'aviary'.

THE RENTOKIL TWINS, SPECKLES AND SQUABBY

As I was hurrying down Terminus Road one morning, there was an extra squash on the pavement where people were gazing upwards at the imposing and bulky Rentokil machinery which was directing its anti-pigeon paraphernalia towards one of the big stores. 'Pigeon trouble' I said to myself. And indeed the next day I had a call from the Veterinary Surgeon; two young pigeons had been brought in. I went to fetch them. The V.S. had done a wonderful job on ungluing them, as far as this was possible, and, of course, there was no proof that the glue was Rentokil, but 'glue' it was. I took the sticky little things and so pathetic and skinny did they look that I put them in a largish cage next to the Dimplex radiator in the bathroom as I was pretty sure they would not wish to roam. This surmise proved correct and they settled happily into the warmth.

They quickly became known as 'the Rentokil twins', though we could not be certain either that they were twins or that their state was actually due to Rentokil. One bird, rather more feathered than the other, we called 'Speckles', while the babyish one we called 'Squabby'. Speckles ate, while Squabby bleeped, so that I had to hand-feed him.

Once again, after a probationary period, and when Squabby started eating on his own, the twins were transferred to the stable aviary. Here Squeaker eyed them suspiciously and awed them into a suitable radius of respect at meal-times. Otherwise all went peacefully.

At a considerably later date when the twins had grown-up and had moulted out of their congealed plumage, Speckles had blossomed into a presentable female. She then excited Squeaker's attentions. These proved acceptable and one morning when Mrs. Rowland (the cleaner already mentioned) asked me, over the Hoover, how my 'family' were doing, I said, 'Fine, thank you; and you know what? Squeaker has married one of the Rentokil twins.' 'You announced *that*,' came the chortling reply, 'just as if it were a society wedding.' I laughed too and could not help thinking how much more engaging the photographs in the *Tatler* might be!

The married couple have moved into the cote vacated by Bertie.

ROSIE

Rosie always put me in mind of the delectable ditty concerning 'Little Polly Perkins of Paddington Green'. Certainly she was 'as bee-u-ti-ful as a butterfly'—she was a Collared Dove, dainty as a Japanese print.

When I fetched her from the surgery the Veterinary Surgeon had told me ruefully how he had gone to great lengths to try and tempt a group of Collared Doves to take up residence in the superb quarters he had provided. Alas, they fled—in search of trees. These exquisite little creatures with their subtle, pearly and lavender colouring suffused with a blush like a reflected sunset, blend in perfectly with the trunks and branches of the trees they love so much.

The first time I heard their strange and unmistakable call, an almost hissed, drawn-out 'oo-oo-oo!' I thought I had come across a daylight owl. A couple of summers ago a little colony of them settled in the trees in the park so that I knew Rosie could ultimately be safely released to join them.

Rosie, presumably, had had a 'bash' of some kind. Her tail was at complete right angles to her body as though it had been wrenched. As the body of these birds is small and no longer than the tail itself, her movement was impeded to such an extent that she preferred to keep still; there was no other visible sign of injury but she could not fly. Unlike the pigeons she was not ravenous.

Rosie started in a basket on its side on the draining-board. Mrs. Rowland on seeing her for the first time exclaimed in delighted admiration. She also commented on her beautiful manners. 'And what on earth does that mean?' I can positively hear the impatient exclamation. Well, she never got agitated or fussed when one was working around the draining-board.

She always excreted very neatly just where one would want her to! She ate happily in an undemanding way, without scattering bits, and drank without upsetting the water. She was generally contented and the minimum of trouble, which is what I mean when I say a student has good manners!

On the second or third day, having watched Rosie's struggles with her uncontrollable tail, and feeling very bold, I fetched the scissors and snipped about one and a half inches off the top ends of the tail-feathers. This brought immediate relief, and the rest of the tail no longer dragged about at right angles. Rosie improved rapidly and was promoted to the bathroom—thence to the open-air aviary. This was equipped with perches and ledges and Rosie strayed uncomfortably among them. I found a good branch and set it up. She took to it immediately.

After about a fortnight Rosie showed signs of restlessness and I wondered whether she could, in fact, fly in spite of her shortened tail. The advantage of the small outside aviary is that it is a wired-off part of a much larger aviary, the latter being unwired at the top and so open to the skies. Any bird released from the smaller inner aviary, and unsure of itself need venture no farther than the larger one (which has a tall elder tree growing in it) and can retire into the smaller one for greater security if so inclined. I, therefore, decided to open the door of the smaller aviary to see what Rosie would do. I had not long to wait. Her flight only a trifle uncertain at first, she made for the nearest oak-tree in the park, and there she rested on a branch, looking absolutely at home. That was the last I saw of her. When I returned to the tree a little later on she was no longer visible. I have no doubt she had joined her fellow-doves in the park.

HEH, NUNNY-NO

This bird was taken to the Veterinary Surgeon's surgery by a nun (hence her name!) There was no visible injury, but the feathers were in a bad state, frayed, with a sticky look. The bird appeared to be in poor condition, very dirty and could not fly. The nun's brother had picked it up in Seaside. When I asked the Veterinary Surgeon's wife, who brought it to me in a box, what colour it was, she said it was grey.

I wanted to try and find out what might be the matter with Heh, Nunny-no, so I put her in a basket in the bathroom. She did not attempt to move and ate modestly. Her droppings were greenish and rather liquid so I put her on a dose of Dianimol once a day for a week and by that time her droppings had become firm and of the normal colour. Hence I suspected that she had had some mild form of enteritis. She ate more and walked about a very little. It also dawned on me that nature had intended her to be white! However it would not have been wise to have bathed her at that stage, though I did so later on. I gave her an adexalin capsule daily to help improve her general state of health. She improved, and always sat docilely on my lap to take her medicine. Finally after about three weeks to a month I put her into the stable aviary with the other pigeons thinking that company might cheer her up. I put her basket, on its side, with a towel over half of the front, into the stable. She tended to stay inside and I put her food in the basket to make sure she got it. Then I noticed she seemed to have some discomfort in walking. I examined her feet and found she had very large, hard pads, like corns on both feet. I took her to the Veterinary Surgeon who told me this condition could be similar to that known as 'Bumblefoot' which was often found in poultry kept in dirty living conditions. No wonder poor Heh, Nunny-no had appeared to be grey! The V.S. gave me some extra strong iodine, and I began to paint her feet with this. She was terribly well-behaved and trustingly let me do anything to her without making the slightest fuss. She would now go out in the yard a little, but she always looked rather depressed and droopy and it made me sad that she seemed not to be making any real progress. I had recently had a bottle of Neomycene sent to me by Mrs. Marsault with the recommendation that this was an excellent general antibiotic which she had found beneficial.

When I had taken Heh, Nunny-no to the Veterinary Surgeon for her 'Bumblefoot' I had told him I was worried at her lack of vitality, so unlike the other pigeons and he had remarked that she might, for all one could tell, be suffering from some obscure sickness or other. I thought the Neomycene might be just the thing to help Heh, Nunny-no to get on top of whatever seemed to be delaying her progress, so I decided to try a small teaspoonful, diluted. I administered this, Heh, Nunny-no swallowing it in meek obedience. To my horror the effect was instantaneous. She gasped, closed her eyes, and leant over sideways. I rushed to get a small blanket, and wrapping it round her placed her in the sun to rest. She never again opened her eyes and died at the end of about forty minutes of semi-consciousness. I was appalled as I had clearly killed her. Yet I was mystified too. The V.S., endlessly patient and helpful as usual, said he would do a post mortem. I took the pathetic little body to the surgery and also the bottle of Neomycene. Later when I rang up the Veterinary Surgeon told me that the post mortem had revealed nothing in the least abnormal, nor was there anything about the bottle of Neomycene that should have been harmful. Mrs. Marsault was equally mystified when I told her about it, and emphatic that the Neomycene could not have done any damage. Nevertheless, I resolved that never again would I use Neomycene. I can only suppose that the dose was too strong for the bird and that I should have diluted it far more. In watching the pigeons I have had since, I also think I was wrong in thinking I could hasten Heh, Nunny-no's convalescence. When a pigeon is *really* in poor condition (as opposed to recuperating from an injury such as a fracture) it takes a very long time to pick up, and only good food, warm clean quarters, rest, spontaneous exercise, and time can really help.

For myself the most painfully distressing thing about Heh, Nunny-no's death was the betrayal of a bird's trust. Sick animals and birds are so utterly defenceless and dependent on the integrity of the human being in whose power they are, that one's responsibility is infinitely great. It is important at all times to diagnose one's own attitude, for frequently the real answer lies there. I decided sadly that this was so in Heh, Nunny-no's case. Behind the genuine desire for her to get well, lay a scratchy seed of impatience which had led me to the fatal experiment. You *cannot* nurse sick birds and allow yourself to grow impatient. I am convinced that had I left her alone to recover in her own good time—and for each patient this is different—she would have been alive now, a healthy and contented bird.

DORCAS

I would like to end these 'cases' with Dorcas. Dorcas was handed over to me by the Raystede Animal Rescue Centre immediately after she had been picked up. Miss Raymonde-Hawkins very kindly telephoned me because she had heard that Binkie, my blackbird, was depressed after losing his guillemot companion and she thought perhaps the injured pigeon might be a suitable substitute. As it turned out Binkie was never very interested in pigeons, largely I suspect because they never evinced any interest in him; but he remains obsessed with a fondness for guillemots and sparrows.

The pigeon was clearly a bathroom bird and got the usual treatment for shock, namely warmth, basket, quiet, water and food. There was no visible injury at first sight, and the pigeon was still partly a squab. The half-grown stage is the most vulnerable for all birds, and pigeons are no exception.

It was a dark day, and the bird seemed sleepy. As I could not see anything I decided to leave the bird alone till next day. I therefore got something of a shock when I placed the pigeon on my knee next morning and lifting its right wing saw that it had a deep and gory gash from top to bottom. This would certainly need stitching. With all speed I took the patient to the surgery. The V.S. corroborated that it would have to be sewn up. I felt guilty at foisting such an extra job on to him. 'Well,' he said quietly, as he deftly removed a blob of dirt and blood from the wound, 'We must do these things; *someone's* got to be humane, and I really think it had better have a general clean-up too.' With admiration and gratitude in my heart I arranged to fetch the pigeon after her 'op' in the evening. She was handed to me by the Veterinary Surgeon's cheerful and competent young assistant, and when I exclaimed at the wonderful job that had been done, and the standard of the 'seam' so to speak, she said, 'He took an *awful* lot of trouble.' This was plain to see, and so to celebrate the needlework the patient was christened 'Dorcas'.

I was much afraid lest Dorcas, who seemed greatly pepped-up might get above herself and perhaps burst a stitch. Hence I quickly gave her a night-cap of a teaspoonful of whisky and water which duly put an end to any untoward activities she might have indulged in. Binkie regarded her somewhat inebriated state with interest, and continued to flit round her basket during the couple of days that she rested in it. Dorcas then became active and exactly a week later she was flying round the yard with the other pigeons. At the time of writing she has shed all signs of 'squabbiness' and has put on a new coat, her wing-feathers having an unusual touch of rose.

There is always a more or less steady trickle of fractures, mostly wing but also leg. One pigeon which was brought in with an injured eye and a broken jaw, was clearly in great pain and was put to sleep.

The Veterinary Surgeon showed me how to strap up the straightforward fractured wings or 'dropped wings' due perhaps to being wrenched or pulled in some way. The birds usually make excellent recoveries and nearly all of them fly again. It is a matter of weeks, sometimes months and some of them, even when they can fly, remain as permanent residents. The gardener counts them from time to time with much head-shaking for he, too, does not approve of 'pampering pigeons'.

I had some difficulty in deciding what to feed the permanent residents on, for they did not much like the standard 'pigeon mixture' or mixed corn sold in the shops. They did, however, rush to eat the 'Swoop' which I scattered for the wild birds. I noticed that they generally made first for the crushed maize, so finally I concocted a mixture of my own, consisting of the wild bird mixture made up and sold locally, which I could buy in bulk, and to which I added extra pounds of crushed maize. I was relieved to find that this seemed to meet the requirements of my very motley collection of pigeons, since 'Swoop' can only be bought in packets and would have proved ruinously expensive. Fortunately I am able to supplement the birds' diet with food from the waste-bin in the College kitchen. The kitchen staff obligingly leave out a bowlful for me every day together with a tin of toast left over from breakfast, and once a day I give them a meal of 'scraps'. I must own that I had no idea that pigeons adore sausages, veal and ham pie, and chopped bacon and ham. I only made this discovery by accidentally dropping some of the bits I was about to throw on to the woodshed roof for the jackdaws. Now the remains of sausage and bacon breakfasts and veal and ham pie suppers are eagerly awaited by the pigeon population.

Apart from their twice—or thrice—daily feeds (according to the weather) the birds wander round the yard eating the milk-thistles sprouting between the bricks, and into a closed-in grassy patch where the laundry is hung out, and where they can peck about freely. The more venturesome spirits go farther afield in the grounds.

Pigeons are fanatical bathers and I have to keep both their shallow bathing bowls plentifully replenished. During the cold spell around Christmas, the caretaker's wife came to tell me in tones of great alarm that one of them had got through the ice on the bowl and was now sitting firmly in the freezing water with lumps of ice clinking around him. It was Greyling (who has since left us) and he never could forego his bath. When I went to look he did not budge and spent the greater part of a very chilly afternoon obstinately refusing to let anyone else share his pleasures! A crestfallen ring of pigeons of varying shapes and sizes roamed frustratedly around him.

'There are none so blind as those that won't see,' says the old adage, and the determined pigeon-exterminator will stick, literally, to his guns and—far worse—to his poisons.

Rachel Carson's awful warning and her magnificent appeal* will go alike unheeded. It would seem appropriate to end this chapter with a thought-provoking quotation from an article by Maitland Edey in *Marvels and mysteries of our Animal*

* *Silent Spring* by Rachel Carson. Published in Great Britain, Hamish Hamilton 1963. Penguin Books 1965.

*World** 'The fate of the passenger pigeon is almost unbelievable. Just a century ago these birds were probably the most numerous on earth. Yet within a span of fifty years human beings succeeded in destroying every last one of them. Nowhere in the long uneven war between men and birds has the rapacity of mankind been so brutally recorded. In 1810 and 1813 flocks with a billion birds to a single flock were observed in Kentucky. In 1914 the last of the pigeons died in the Cincinnati Zoo and is now stuffed and to be seen in the Smithsonian Institution in Washington. (They ate acorns and beechnuts.)'

* Coronet Books. The Reader's Digest Association. Pleasantville, New York.

CHAPTER EIGHT

Guillemots

(Post Torrey Canyon)

My husband once confessed to me that when a little boy, he had thought that nuns were penguins, never having met one of the latter. I, too, had childhood visions of penguins, though of a more secular nature. I longed to have one for a friend. It is odd how often such wishes are granted if you wait long enough, though the capricious Genie who deals us these favours usually sees to it that neither the manner nor the moment is of our own choosing.

So it happened that one tempestuous day in January of 1968, while on a duty-walk along the sea-front my eye was caught by a flint-coloured heap performing spasmodic movements just beyond the wave-limit. I rushed down the slope to find, at the bottom a harassed-looking woman in a green mackintosh who was gazing at the heap. 'Can you help me?' I yelled above the wind as I lowered myself on to the beach and climbed over the groyne. Exasperatingly, the heap was not on a beach with steps. The good woman obediently started to manoeuvre the obstacles. Inspired by zeal, and alas, by ignorance, I stumbled rapidly towards the heap which I had identified as guillemot and which to my inexperienced eyes seemed far too exhausted to be capable of any effort. I was, therefore, startled when, as I approached, the bird seemed to collect its last scraps of strength and as the wave licked up towards it, staggered into the spray—I followed; too late—it was on the crest of the next wave but one.

In a flash I realised my folly. (It was some weeks later that I read Tony Soper's warning remark in *The Wreck of the Torrey Canyon*, 'first catch your bird'.) Frustrated and furious with myself I turned to face my aide, now perched on the groyne. 'I reported that to the R.S.P.C.A. an hour ago,' she said, and as if in response to the rubbing of a magic lamp, the Inspector hove in sight above us, complete with basket. 'I've muffed it,' I said. 'How are you going to get out of there?' he replied. I nodded towards the groyne where I had thrown down my purse and the dog's lead. I scrambled back and looked out to sea, where a tiny and receding figure bobbed in the waves, every now and then frantically preening. 'It'll be back with the tide in an hour or two,' the Inspector said reassuringly, seeing my distress. 'Then I'll wait,' I said. 'I have to go to a funeral,' he said gloomily and unexpectedly, and departed. 'I'll come back after lunch,' said the green woman, and departed too. There was no one else in sight.

My bedraggled collie looked at me beseechingly. Inwardly seething, and with my eyes on the distant speck, now rapidly drifting towards Holywell, I started my bleak patrol. It began to sleet icily; I had not expected to be out for longer than half an hour and was wearing a thin nylon rain-cape. At the end of an hour the barely visible speck disappeared, rose again, disappeared, rose and disappeared for good. My dog stubbornly sat down and howled. The sleet hissed past my ears. Well, I'd learnt a lesson—the hard way, as usual. 'All right,' I said to the dog, 'Let's go.'

We paddled dejectedly through the puddles. I was about to turn up towards the pine-trees when something duck-like in the sea making for the shore made me look again. I began to think the cold was causing me to have hallucinations, but it was unmistakably a guillemot. 'Right,' I said to myself, 'I shall put into practice what I have learnt. This time, dear Guillie, you *don't* commit suicide.' The bird staggered out of the water and lay down; then, in short laps, it tottered as far as it could go, and came to rest below me, against the sea wall, and, conveniently this time, to the right of a flight of steps.

I waited another hour; waited for the turning tide to go out so that the space between the bird and the water would allow me to cut it off from its last desperate dive. Even then, at the end of that time, it was clear that I could not safely approach it; a wait of at least another two hours would be necessary. My heart failed me. I thought of getting help, and employing cunning. I returned to the car with my dejected and dripping collie and drove back to College. There I collected an aged shrimping-net I had observed in one of the stables, and two gardeners. Thus equipped and fortified I arrived at the top of the steps and peered over. I was again struck by the incredible camouflage of the guillemots on the flint, but now I knew what to look for. My bird was still there. 'Well,' said one of the gardeners, 'let's have a go,' and took a step down the ladder. 'Oh *don't*.' I let out an agonised appeal but he had already descended two more steps and the bird was in the sea, paddling wearily outwards. There was nothing to be done. I took the gardeners back and drove through the thick sea-mist and murk to my own cottage in the country, but with iron determination in my heart. Some premonition made me stop at a fish-shop. They had no sprats so I was forced to buy coley. I had a feeling that the bird would return to the shore. It was not quite as all-in as the other one had been.

My good neighbour who was looking out of her front window called me as I drew up, 'Whatever have you been doing? You look simply frozen.' 'I *am* frozen; I've been fishing for guillemots,' I said. 'Well, come in and have a glass of rum.' I thankfully accepted the offer and then retreated into my own lair. I rubbed down my patient, long-suffering dog with a warm towel, put some soup on the stove, and fished in the airing-cupboard for pullovers and trousers. It was almost dark; by the time I had donned three layers, top and bottom, and had drunk the soup, it was quite dark. The tide must be well out by now. With gratitude in my heart for the imaginative student who had presented me with a powerful Pifco for Christmas, I started off. I parked the car at a favourite point on the empty promenade and set off with shrimping-net and Pifco. The tide was out beyond the ends of the groynes. I sent the strong beam of light across the first beach and on to the rocks beyond; nothing. The second beach; nothing. The third beach, empty. I flashed the light to and fro, and suddenly a minute black and white penguin-like figure arose in the middle of the sandy patch and signalled with its small bent arms. Then it collapsed. It was on a beach with no stairs. I rushed down the parallel beach, turned the groyne and slowed down. I could see the little black and white lump motionless on the sand without the torch. One would have thought it was just another of the many stones strewn around by the retreating tide. As I came up to it, it attempted to hoist itself to its feet and took a longitudinal lurch towards the sea, but this time the odds were heavily on my side. I popped the shrimping-net over it, inserted my hand underneath and grasped the clammy cold little body. It struggled feebly, but when I picked it up and placed it against my hairy Norwegian ski-jacket, it sank peacefully against the soft material.

Once at the cottage, I dried the little creature as well as I could with a towel and put it in front of the fire, in a basket on its side. It wriggled out of the basket towards the fire and lay down on the hearthrug, flicked its wings and looked round with contentment in its eye.

I fetched the coley, cut it into strips and presented these. It was not interested, shut its eyes and promptly fell asleep, not in any way put out by sharing the hearthrug with the collie. I felt strongly inclined to follow its example so made my way upstairs with some steaming coffee, and, I suspect, a degree of contentment in my eye too.

Nevertheless sprats kept swimming in and out of my slumbers and the next morning, after another fruitless effort with the coley, I started operation sprats. 'Out of season, out of season, no ma'am out of season.' It was like a Gilbert and Sullivan refrain.

Although it was holiday time, I was forced to go to College that day to interview candidates applying for the post of assistant matron. I naturally could not leave my guillemot unattended at the cottage, so he had perforce to come with me, in the cat-basket used on such occasions. He settled down comfortably in the basket, and at College I deposited him on the hearthrug by the electric fire in my room. I had bought a herring on the way, and after de-boning it, I cut it into narrow two-inch strips and waggled these before him without exciting any interest. I tried force-feeding but he obstinately spewed up the strips. After telephoning Mrs. Marsault I let him drink fresh, cold water out of a cup (to 'keep the kidneys going', Mrs. Marsault had said) and pushed half a tablet of Vitamin B down his throat. It stayed down. After this he lay down on the rug and went to sleep, with his head turned to the right on to his back and his beak resting in the groove between the wings.

Interviewing members of that migratory species seeking a comfortable roost, preferably with centrally-heated perch, as school or college matron, is guaranteed to liquidate all but super-human confidence and optimism. It was a relief to turn once more to the sanity of birds. The guillemot slept peacefully, but I *must* get sprats. Mrs. Marsault had said so.

I started to telephone along the coast. Finally a friend knew a friend who knew a fisherman. By 1.30 p.m., breakfastless and lunchless we had located Uncle Tom's Cabin in Hastings Old Town, reputed to have received sprats from Kent that day. It was pouring and the sky was black. There was an occasional roll of thunder as the car splashed along the Hastings road. A matey youngster emerged from the misty depths of Uncle Tom's Cabin, and confirmed that he had a box of sprats. I said I would take the box and he disappeared behind the Cabin to re-emerge a few minutes later, odorous box in hand. He evinced interest in the guillemot project, though remarking that they were 'vicious birds' and he promised to deliver more sprats, a promise which never materialised. Elated, I drove back in a state of high sprat-euphoria, stopping only to collect some Fuller's Earth at a chemist for a preliminary dry de-oiling.

Arrived at the cottage, having collected my bird from College, I lost no time in extracting a handful of sprats from the box and placing these before a moderately interested guillemot. He lay once more upon the cottage hearth-rug, and cocked a languid eye at the sprats as they gleamed before him. I went back into the kitchen to forestall any unintended sprat-consumers from foraging. A neighbour had recently acquired an exploratory cat. I put the sprats in a safe place and returned to the guillemot. There were two sprats only; I had put down five. I felt too excited to feel certain. I fetched more sprats, and then for the first time I watched how a guillemot skilfully and infallibly got his sprat down head-first. He had nine sprats in a row and then paused with a satisfied flick of wings and tail. I had no idea how many sprats a guillemot would eat at one sitting or even in one day. I had nothing to go on and nothing to compare with. I thought of sitting down myself to a supper of nine grilled sprats, and thought of prisoners-of-war existing on a handful of rice a day and decided it was not too bad.

Then I had my own compound meal of the day by the fire, intelligently watched by 'Janni'. I had already decided to call him this to remind myself that he was rescued in the month of January, actually on Thursday, 4th January (1968).

So that was how I acquired my first charming and gentle guillemot. He did not appear badly oiled—indeed I suspected that he had already been amateurishly 'de-oiled' and had been disastrously 'released' as he was obviously not waterproof. Since he was also very exhausted, and thin, I merely mopped off surplus oil (*dry* oil, i.e. not the thick, pitchy, sticky stuff) with Fuller's earth. He enjoyed this and co-operatively held out his wing so that I could rub underneath. After that I did no more till I got back to College, as I felt the important thing was for him to recover his strength. While still at the college he ate sprats happily, rested by the fire, was interested in all that went on around him and slept well, with his head cosily cradled between his wings as on the first day.

Janni was rescued on *4th January*.

On *5th January* in the evening he had his first meal of nine sprats.

On *6th January* I heard him moving at 6.30 a.m. and his food programme was as follows:

6.30 a.m.	2 sprats.
7.30 a.m.	2 sprats.
8.30 a.m.	1 sprat plus ½ tablet Vitamin B pushed into sprat's stomach, through slit made with point of knife.
	1 sprat during morning, while I was out.
1.30 p.m.	2 sprats.

3.00 p.m. 1 sprat.
5.30 p.m. 1 sprat.
7.00 p.m. 1 sprat.
10.00 p.m. 1 sprat just before I went to bed.
Total 13 sprats

Janni spent two more days at the cottage, totalling 12 sprats on 7th January and only eight on Monday, 8th January.

On 9th January I left the cottage to return to College in preparation for the coming term. It was a freezing, snowy day and at College I put Janni in the bathroom where he rapidly got the hang of the Dimplex radiator. From then on one of his favourite spots was on a towel, placed over a square of sponge rubber (obtainable at Woolworth's) standing close up to the radiator as though he were facing a warm rock in his natural environment. I soon realised that the front-against-the-wall attitude must be characteristic. The guillemots that followed Janni, when they were well enough to stand, all automatically turned to the wall or some upstanding object; in my case always the radiator. Later I read somewhere that guillemots in their colonies face the rock, with their black backs toning in with it, and only turn their white fronts round when alerted of something.

By this time I had established over the telephone to Mrs. Marsault, that in her experience also, her oiled guillemots frequently did not eat more than two sprats at one go, and averaged roughly eleven sprats a day, though this varied. I felt a good deal easier in my mind after this conversation, as just how many sprats a guillemot ought to consume is a burning question when you have got one, and certainly no bird-book tells you. Matron had already fallen hook, line and sinker a victim to the guillemot personality and as both she and I were interested in the odd variation of sprat-consumption, which seemed as erratic as a typhoid-chart, Matron made a sprat-chart from my records for each guillemot. (See Appendix III). They also show when certain 'medicines' or vitamins were given. I would have given much to have had such a chart available at the time when I spent sleepless nights, worrying myself sick about the unpredictable variations in sprat-'temperature'.

Meanwhile Janni became increasingly affectionate, and when I went up to my room after the evening lesson, I used to fetch him from the bathroom and he sat on my lap, reclining cosily, rather like a kitten, while I did my corrections. Before long I merely used to open the bathroom door, and out he waddled to the hearth-rug in my room waiting for me to sit down in the armchair when he would hold out his arms ready to be picked up and placed on my lap. On Sunday, 14th January, he 'talked' for the first time, a curious kind of squawk; he did this three times. His sprat-consumption was down and I was getting very worried, especially as I was encountering all kinds of unsuspected difficulties in getting sprats. One shop which had sworn by all that was holy that they always kept a stock of sprats in the deep freeze, I need not worry, then said sorry, they had sold the lot when I went to get some. Matron and I spent a great deal of time exploring the fish-shops of Eastbourne, Hailsham and Battle to keep Janni's supply going. It soon became apparent that they had to be very fresh or he would not eat them. Finally the College chef kindly came to my rescue by allowing me to use a corner of his deep freeze to store sprats, so that when we did see them in the shops we could lay in several pounds. For some inexplicable reason, the assistants serving in fish-shops seemed to have their worst instincts aroused by any request for more than two pounds of sprats. Already at two pounds their eyebrows would shoot up and as if talking to a mentally retarded customer they would say, in a disciplinary tone of voice: 'ONE pound of sprats?' 'No, *two* pounds, please.' 'That's a lot of fish, you know?' they would go on, and if kindly disposed they would add 'dear!' 'Yes, I know, I *love* grilled sprats; *must* make the most of the season,' I would say summoning my most obsequious smile. But FOUR pounds of sprats was no longer a laughing matter. Matron was, on the whole much better at it than I was. I invariably excited suspicion. Anyhow we always reported to each other any new batch of sprats and then went in separately leaving a decent interval for the assistant to recover in.

I once made a fatal error, never to be lived down, by confiding to the assistant the real destination of the fish. Thereafter, as soon as he spotted me at the counter, he would put on a ferocious glare and bellow 'You're the one that buys all them sprats for *birds*.' He always managed to make it sound as if this were an anti-social act of the first magnitude or as if I were depriving India's starving millions of their only hope of salvation. The effect was so undermining that I nearly always came out with a pound less than I had intended, so that poor Matron had to make up for my deficiencies.

Janni did not like his fish limp. He liked them icy cold, and although both Dorothy Yglesias and Mrs. Marsault had told me not to bother to get sea-water to present them in—their guillemots ate them just as happily out of a shallow dish of ordinary cold tap-water—I found that Janni was less obliging and definitely preferred his sprats in, or just out of, salt water. I tried putting salt into ordinary tap-water, but this was an utter failure. I put too much or too little and was everlastingly licking sample teaspoonsful and finding them awful as did Janni. It was far easier to go to the beach and fill one of the gallon plastic containers which had held orange juice. This lasted a good while and I had no more bother. Actually Janni preferred being hand fed, and rarely touched any fish which had been left lying near him. He used to follow up his sprat-swallowing with much head-shaking and drops of moisture used to come from his nostrils. This also alarmed me, as I thought he had perhaps caught cold and would contract the deadly pneumonia. I paid him several visits at 3 a.m. to make sure he was warm enough, but always found him cuddled up against the Dimplex radiator, and apparently comfortable. Later, experience taught me that all guillemots (or, at least, those I had) shook their heads after eating and exuded moisture from their nostrils, though in varying degrees.

Dorothy Yglesias had generously given me a tin of Tremalon when I was in Mousehole after the disaster of the *Torrey Canyon*, in case I might need it. She had realised only too clearly that from now on oiled guillemots would be on the increase and would spread, though she and her sister had dealt with them for about thirty years, uttering warnings which had gone unheeded. Nowhere had anyone had more experience over a longer period of years, and now I rejoiced to have a de-oiling agent recommended by her.

On Sunday, 28th January, Matron and I drew a deep breath and for the first time in our lives attempted to de-oil a guillemot. We were fortunate indeed for we had the best stuff to do it with; our bird was not badly oiled, and we had only one. Even so, speaking for myself, I was in a state of awful trepidation. It was a lovely sunny morning, and we began our operations at about 10 a.m. We put Janni on a large square of fibreboard placed across the bath and while Matron held his head so that nothing could get into his eyes, I worked the Tremalon into his feathers, stroking always *with* the feathers and *never* against them, as Dorothy Yglesias had previously told me to do. Matron had already prepared four large bowls of very lukewarm water, and also the hand-basin. We rinsed Janni in all of them in turn, and finally in the bath itself. He was mortally alarmed by the water, but responded quickly to being dried in hot towels which he clearly liked, and then after a spell in front of the electric fire he sat in the sun on the sponge-rubber I had spread on the cushions of the window-seat. He ate a sprat which I offered him and greatly enjoyed the sunshine, looking out of the window, and preening his clean feathers. The previous Sunday (21st January) he had reached his record number of sprats in a day, totalling 16. Whether his bath affected his appetite or not I do not know, but he ate only two more sprats that day, one at 5.30 p.m. and one before he went to bed. He was lively, however, and I was beginning to control my anxiety at these unaccountable fluctuations.

From now on Janni, de-oiled, serene in his daily routine, led a tranquil existence. He had the run of the bathroom, though he stayed at the Dimplex end from choice, and as guillemots, like other sea-birds, excrete prolifically, I automatically mopped up the linoleum every time I came in.

In February, however, a change came into his life—and mine. I was now drawn like a magnet to the beach, especially to a certain groyne, where I had often seen the R.S.P.C.A. Inspector patrolling. Hence on Thursday, 8th February, I was once again walking my dog along the front, when I spotted the now familiar struggling lump on the edge of the wave-line. A young man had spotted it too and was making motions as if to approach. Knowing how catastrophic this would be, I shouted to him, and slithered down through the bushes on to the lower concrete parade. 'Please,' I called out, 'don't move. That's an oiled guillemot. Please stay and watch it, while I run and get my net.' The young man was friendly but said what anybody would have done in his place, 'All right, but it looks all-in to me. Are you sure it can move?' 'Pretty sure,' I said, and fled for the net in my car. I rushed back with it to find young man and guillemot still in place. This time, having learnt my lesson, I cautiously walked into the sea at some distance from the bird. I was wearing wellingtons, but as the bird had not had the strength to stagger far out of the water I was forced to wade out up to my knees in order to cut it off. As I worked my way inwards towards the bird, it panicked and lunged towards the sea. Fortunately I was anticipating this, and was able to drop the shrimping-net over it. It struggled and I held the net down till the young man who at the start of the operation had clearly decided I had taken leave of my senses, joined me, saying 'And you were right about that bird. I'd never have believed it.' He obligingly now held the net, while I inserted my hand and came out with a sodden, terrified, and furiously fighting guillemot. I held the bird against my jacket but hanging on to him firmly. The young man hooked the net over my shoulder and with water bubbling over the tops of my wellington boots, I squelched back to the car, while another interested onlooker remarked, 'I thought there weren't any oiled sea-birds any more.' It was already 4 p.m., and I had to teach at 4.15 p.m. As soon as I got to College, I towelled the slightly calmer guillemot and not daring to put him with Janni, I left him in the warm kitchen in the corner by the cupboard under the sink—the cupboard beloved of Jack Devon, the jackdaw. I swept out the contents of the bottom ground-level shelf and left the sliding door half-open. Then I discovered I was clamped into my wellingtons and had to find someone to pull me out of them, leaving a trail of frothy little puddles all along the corridor in the process. Finally I arrived in the classroom on the dot of 4.15 p.m. with spectacular purple weals all over my hands and wrists and a few damp patches still about my person.

At the end of the lesson I shot upstairs to find the guillemot on the floor beside the cupboard. I suspected his legs were too bad for him to negotiate the slight 'step' into it. I pushed a Dianimol capsule down his throat and had to be content with that, as he resisted with whatever strength he had left.

Matron came up to inspect him, and I told her of my decision to call him Mr. Kwak out of respect for the Dutchman of that unlikely name who had come over to Mousehole to help with the victims of the *Torrey Canyon.*

Mr. Kwak was much larger and *broader* than Janni who always gave the impression of being tall and slim. This was partly because he now stood a good deal, and was well up on his toes. Poor Mr. Kwak was very weak on the legs, and immediately collapsed whenever he attempted to hoist himself on to his feet. He had a curiously humped look like a slightly hunch-backed human being would have had. He too, had obviously been 'de-oiled' and indiscriminately released, for he had next to no oil visible except for a very little under the wings. It had certainly not all been preened off, because he was not excreting jets of pure oil as did those badly oiled but half-preened birds I subsequently came in contact with. He was utterly exhausted and like a wet dish-rag; not the slightest bit waterproof.

At 1 a.m. bothered by his refusal to touch any food I force-fed him one sprat. It stayed down.

At 7.15 a.m. the next day, Friday 9th February, I gave another Dianimol capsule and at 11.15 a.m. an adexalin bobble. (These capsules are red and round and often given to children. Mrs. Marsault had put me on to them.) He resolutely refused fish and at 4.15 p.m. I administered another adexalin. He looked better, was less frightened which meant he did not wear himself out threshing about on the floor as soon as I appeared, and by the evening he even managed to stand a little. I tried to force-feed him sprats but these he regurgitated every time. At 10 p.m. I fed him half a tablet of Vitamin B. He would not drink out of a cup as Janni had done.

On Saturday, 10th February, I gave him one Dianimol and one adexalin capsule at 7 a.m. I also force-fed a small bit of liver containing half a tablet of Vitamin B. He continued to refuse food. At 7 p.m. that night I again force-fed one adexalin capsule and one bit of liver. I was just able to push the liver down and as it was very small and slippery it was not brought up again.

On Sunday I knew I must do something desperate to make him eat. At 7 a.m. he had two bits of liver and half a tablet of Vitamin B and he kept down the tail end of a sprat. At 8.15 a.m. to my great joy he ate, of his own accord, *three* sprats. After that it was plain sailing and by the evening he had totalled 14 sprats. From then on there was no more difficulty in feeding Mr. Kwak. He also took up residence in the kitchen cupboard on that Sunday. Shortly after that I decided that in view of his apparently uncontaminating state, I could safely put him in the bathroom with Janni. Janni was cautious but was soon won over by Mr. Kwak's jolly sociability. The two birds were of totally different temperaments. Janni was gentle, reserved and affectionate. Mr. Kwak, once over his initial terror, was jovial in the extreme, rumbustious, almost in the joyous appreciation of his convalescence. Janni was slightly wistful at missing his evening sessions on my lap. I had not the heart to exclude Mr. Kwak from these sessions, yet my lap would only accommodate one guillemot at a time, and time was precious. I thought as the two birds had each other's company they could now entertain each other. Janni never lost his slight clinging to human company, and when the time came I found it hard to part with him. Mr. Kwak was an unabashed extrovert who found everything rather a lark, and never made a fuss, even when suffering wretched discomforts on account of his weak and unsupporting legs. I must confess I found it just as hard to part with him, but I felt he would console himself more easily and adapt more readily to new surroundings.

In the meantime, while still much concerned with Mr. Kwak, I received another addition to the guillemot family. As soon as I had received the telephone call, I rushed round to fetch the bird. It turned out to be very small and badly oiled. I fetched it on Saturday, 10th February, the day before Mr. Kwak began to eat. The new bird was in a daunting mess; fresh, sticky, pitchy oil covered the breast and all the underparts. Its comparative smallness made us call it the Mini-guillie straight away. It was bright-eyed, but it was impossible to postpone the de-oiling. I fetched the bird at 5 p.m. and after giving it the routine Dianimol capsule to clear its intestines of oil, Matron and I set to work on the de-oiling. It was the first 'REAL' job we had had. At the end of it, a good deal of the oil had been transferred to our persons, but our bird was certainly cleaner. After her bath she drank a lot and ate four sprats. We always called her 'she' regardless of our ignorance of guillemot sex.

I visited her during the night and she ate two more sprats. As she was not yet entirely without oil, I had put her in the kitchen and not with Janni. She rapidly discovered Mr. Kwak in the kitchen cupboard, invaded his quarters and was effusively and delightedly all over him. He did not relish these attentions, but later when he tried to escape from them, Mini pursued him with persistence, and when the three birds were finally united in the bathroom, she was equally demonstrative towards Janni who was visibly embarrassed. Indeed this 'running after the boys' as we used to call it, proved to be her undoing in the end, for she came between a mating pair at the Exmouth hospital and got severely pecked on the head for her interference. From this punishment she did not recover, in spite of the devoted attention bestowed upon her by Mrs. Marsault, and we all grieved deeply.

On Sunday, the day after she arrived, we were disturbed at the amount of oil still left on Mini, and with great misgivings gave her another Tremalon bath, followed by a first rinse in a bucket of warm water containing three squirts of Fairy liquid. The oil poured out of her feathers at this point and after her four subsequent rinses in pure warm water finishing up in the actual bath itself, she looked very much better. Hot towels were ready, and once she was dry, we concentrated on restoring her strength and appetite, although she had not refused food from the beginning. She ate eight sprats on that Sunday, on top of the three she had eaten during the night. She still drank a good deal and with great eagerness. I was pleased about this, as I hoped it would help to clear out her internal intake of the oil. Normally guillemots do not appear to drink as they presumably get their liquid through the fish. This, of course, I did not know. Certainly some oiled guillemots are grateful for fresh water, though as they get better so their interest in drinking grows less. Others, like Mr. Kwak, do not seem to drink at all.

Ménage à trois.

From the time all three guillemots were together in the bathroom a certain routine became established.

My bathroom is long and narrow and though the birds were never confined, they mostly kept to one end in the vicinity of the larger of the two Dimplex radiators. The smaller one is by the window at the opposite end and as it is attached to the wall they could not cuddle up to it as they did with the other one, whenever they felt chilly. Next to the radiator is a recess for hanging clothes. They all adored this dark cave and I lined the floor with sheets of sponge rubber which I changed and washed out daily. This was a very simple task, as the droppings came off easily in the warm water. The sponge rubber in front of the radiator I covered with an old towel for further warmth and comfort. I also placed a couple of cardboard boxes on their sides on the floor. They were just over the height of a guillemot and with flaps, so they formed a kind of private annexe to the recess, and often one or other of the birds, usually Janni, when overcome by Mini's caresses, would shuffle in for a quiet snooze. I lined these with sponge rubber too, as one of the worst problems arising out of the guillemots' long convalescence is foot and leg trouble. It must be remembered that guillemots are ocean birds and at no time in their normal lives would they support the weight of their bodies on their legs uninterruptedly for months, while their feet were contacting only hard, unyielding surfaces. We oiled their feet and rubbed their legs, first with Vaseline and then with an ointment recommended by Mrs. Marsault. This helped a lot, but Mini's webbing split in more than one place and frayed, while poor Mr. Kwak, who arrived with leg trouble, had a difficult time, though nothing daunted his good spirits. Janni, fortunately, never developed leg trouble but he was the lightest of all three, which possibly had some bearing on the matter. Even little Mini was heavier. Their weights were as follows:

Janni	1 lb.	4	oz.
Mr. Kwak	1 lb.	13-14	oz.
Mini	1 lb.	8	oz.

Once in the swing, the routine was more or less like this:

7 a.m. I gave each guillemot *a sprat* containing a red adexalin capsule. Then I had a cup of tea myself! The guillies were usually together in the clothes recess at this hour and still sleepy.

After my cup of tea, or else after breakfast, I changed their towel and sponge rubber sheets, and washed the dirty ones. There was no actual need to dry these after squeezing the water out of them, as the damp ones were good for their feet. They now had another *sprat* (hand-fed) and then they emerged to line up by the radiator. At break-time, another *sprat*; before lunch, *a sprat*; during the afternoon, *one or two sprats*; before supper, *a sprat*; after supper, *a sprat*, and maybe later on, another *sprat*. These were all hand-fed to make sure everybody was eating the basic minimum, which I put at 8 *sprats* a day—as an average. Of course, frequently they ate more, and the exact records are shown on the charts at the end of the chapter. I also gave a little extra Vitamin B; this again is shown on the charts. I left extra sprats either in a shallow dish of water (which they never seemed to touch) or scattered on the towel—and these they sometimes ate.

All three birds loved human company. After College Assembly, when I was teaching, one of the College cleaners came to clean my quarters. She is an exceptional and endearing person, Sussex-born and country-bred, and she used to visit the guillies and talk to them; or else in the course of her duties she was working in the bathroom. The guillies loved this and would turn inquisitive beaks in her direction; indeed their concerted linear action reminded one of the frieze-like effect of a well-trained corps de ballet.

In the afternoons they tended to have a siesta, but the highlight of their day was when I had finished teaching and came upstairs at five or six o'clock.

I had arranged a wooden box on the window-seat of a south window in my room (also covered in sponge rubber) so that when the guillemots were on it they could look out of the window into the park. As soon as I came upstairs after my evening teaching, I opened the bathroom door, and triumphantly the triumvirate would burst forth—Janni first; then Mini, and last, valiantly trying to keep up with them on his rickety pins Mr. Kwak, helping himself along with his wings. They navigated the rough mat at the entrance to my room, turned right past the back of the couch, occasionally stumbled over the paws of my recumbent collie, and halted with military precision before the window-seat. It was far too high for them to mount alone, so they waited till I lifted them on to the box. There they viewed the scene below, preened themselves and each other (Mini was always busily preening one or other of 'the boys'), ate a sprat or two, and after twenty minutes grew restless and if not lifted down, would attempt to 'fly' down, landing with a thump on the wooden floor. As this was very bad for their feet and legs, I was always on the alert to forestall this unnerving performance, but Mini enjoyed it, and whenever she managed to elude my gaze, she flopped down, and then extended her wings looking towards me mischievously in anticipation of being replaced on the box. When it was 'time ladies and gentlemen', and I had lifted them down they all marched solemnly back to the bathroom, ate a sprat, and began to settle down for the night.

Mini always hopefully squeezed in between Mr. Kwak and Janni, and when Janni tended to detach himself she clung to the broad-bosomed Mr. Kwak.

On Saturdays and Sundays, if it was a sunny morning the window-drill was enhanced by a 'sprinkle-bath'. I would let the birds sun themselves on the box; then they were duly 'watered' with a small watering-can with a fine sprinkle nozzle. This led them to preen and they greatly enjoyed their shower. As they were not in the least waterproof it was too early even to let them swim in the bath. The 'wetness' of their non-waterproof plumage can be clearly seen in the photograph which shows the birds just after their sprinkle-bath. All three wear their characteristic expressions. Nearest the streaming window-panes, slightly hump-backed, is Mr. Kwak, gazing upwards expecting more fun. In front of him, Janni of the grave and thoughtful eye; behind him, and seemingly larger only because of being nearer the camera, Mini, looking, as usual, towards the boys.

One afternoon, sometime during this period, I had gone over to my cottage to do a few hours' gardening. Whenever I was out for any length of time, Matron generously deputised for me, and I would leave sprats for the birds' next feed. If I did happen to snatch a free afternoon I usually came back in time to give the birds their window-seat outing. On this occasion I was a little later than usual though it was a light and sunny evening. As soon as I came in I went straight to the bathroom, but found the door ajar and—to my horror—the bathroom empty. Heart in mouth, I rushed into my sitting-room which was plentifully spattered with guillemot excretions, leading joyfully away from the unsurmountable box-in-window seat to the one at the other end of the wall, with the same view, but without the box, and there, in their usual formation, sat the three escapees, serenely gazing out of the window. They turned their heads as I came in with a look of 'It's all right; we've managed by ourselves, thank you,' in their quiet unperturbed eyes. I felt almost sick with relief and laughed aloud.

They had clearly first essayed to reach their usual look-out but frustrated there and not to be baulked, they had managed to flap and climb on to the lower, parallel one.

The bathroom door-handle is awkward, and occasionally springs open, which is what had given the enterprising trio their opportunity.

Thus the days—as far as the guillemots were concerned—passed peacefully enough. Then the evenings lengthened and whiffs of spring came through the window.

Occasionally, it seemed to me, the birds were restless. I let them have brief swims in the bath, although, of course, they were by no means waterproof.* The Mini-guillie quite enjoyed these sprees as long as the paddle was not prolonged. The other two were thrown into a panic by the water, and flapped frantically against the sides of the bath, so that they had to be lifted out almost immediately. All three were dried on hot towels, and then they sat in the sun on the window-seat. I never put them in the bath if the weather was dull, and never oftener than once a week, nor did I do this till roughly six weeks after I had acquired them.

As the weather grew milder I began to feel the birds ought to be out in the fresh air but I had no pen. I did borrow a sort of portable wire netting pen (about 6 feet by 3 feet) from the gardeners and put the birds in it on the lawn, but they hated it, and cuddled together looking miserable, so after two attempts I gave it up.

However, the Easter holiday was approaching and something would have to be done. I telephoned Mrs. Marsault, most patient and long-suffering of souls, and asked if she could possibly take on three more guillemots. I had seen her guillemots disporting ing themselves in their pool on the grass in their open-air run, with draught-proof night-shelter attached. To my inexpressible relief, she agreed, although she was, in fact, heavily burdened with an outsize batch of fresh guillemots, many of them requiring constant nursing and attention.

I, therefore, arranged to take them down to Exmouth one weekend near the end of term, leaving College on Saturday, spending the night with the Marsaults and returning on the Sunday. The next problem was *how* to transport them. My car is a Morris Traveller, bought second-hand through the kind offices of the garage owner in the village where I have my cottage. When he first telephoned to let me know that he had a second-hand car for sale and I enquired whether it was one suited to my pursuits, a resigned voice replied 'I guess so; there's

* In the experience of those who had charge of the birds of the *Torrey Canyon*, a period of anything from 6 to 12, or even 18 months, is needed before the birds regain their natural oils so as to render them waterproof. Any glib statements concerning quick release and quick re-waterproofing should be regarded as unreliable and dangerous.

plenty of room for your dog, your plants, your *birds*—and your ROCKS!' This last was a scathing allusion to my hobby of pebble-collecting!

I now realise with that clarity attained only in retrospection, that my approach to guillemot transport was more than a little tinged with romanticism. I envisaged the birds happily enthroned at the back of the Traveller, intelligently taking in and enjoying, with their customary enthusiasm, the kaleidescopic sights of English town and country planning in the place of the more static sights of the Park. I, therefore, padded the back of the car with sponge rubber and towels, making what looked to me like a guillemots' Pullman. As I was adding the finishing touches the night before departure, it did seem to me over-illuminated, rather like a conservatory, and I had a mild qualm or two, since, the guillemots, on the whole preferred a soft light and dim corners. At the last moment, therefore, I sorted out two cardboard boxes, lined these also, and placed them in the garage as a reserve, should the Pullman prove unacceptable. There was now a fourth guillemot to be accommodated which the Veterinary Surgeon had brought me two days previously. It had been beautifully de-oiled at the Surgery, looked fat and comfortable (hence christened 'Bulgy') and settled in well with the others.

My assistant matron was coming with me as map-reader, and keeper of the gigantic Thermos containing chilled sprats. My collie was travelling somewhat restrictedly on the back seat. As he often got wedged between articles such as a deck-chair and a Christmas tree, or a selection of objects resembling the sculpture of the sixties, he bore all confinement with stoical endurance, swaying offendedly as he kept a precarious balance on the edge of the seat.

At 7 a.m., with the whole College still mercifully asleep, all were aboard and we set off. Instant uproar ensued. I gritted my teeth and squinted at my passenger who, with sphinx-like expression, was gazing through the windscreen. After about a quarter-of-a-mile I stopped the car and said 'This is hopeless. We'd better go back and try the cardboard boxes.' 'Well, I didn't like to say anything, but I'm most relieved you think so,' said my companion with admirable control.

I went to the back of the car and righted the Mini-guillie who was inverted behind a towel, and tried to soothe Janni and Mr. Kwak who looked as though they had spent several sleepless nights on the British railways. Another idiocy to repent of, I thought dejectedly, and hopped into my seat.

I put the three foundation members, Janni, Mr. Kwak and the Mini-guillie in the large rectangular box with flaps, which left them warm and in the dark while letting in plenty of air. They at once settled down. Bulgy, the newcomer, I put by himself in the blanketed cat-basket, and he too settled into the soft material.

We set off once more. Peace and quiet reigned.

About two hours later we stopped to eat our breakfast sandwiches and drink hot coffee. I visited the back of the car and was met by three enquiring beaks at the top of the box saying plainly in guillemot language 'What about our sandwiches?' I extracted sprats from the Thermos and they were courteously received. After the usual head-shaking which marks post sprat-consumption, beaks were lowered and all was quiet. Bulgy had his sprat in solitude but did not seem to mind.

After another hour or so's driving we suddenly heard a chorus of mild squawks from the cardboard box. Wondering slightly, I went to see what could be disturbing them. Their attitude expressed that they were ready for their elevenses. This they immediately got. From then on, whenever they decided it was time for another sprat they would 'ring the bell' for service.

When we arrived at the Marsault's birds' hospital, the travellers emerged from their receptacles in good trim, to be received into the Marsault's hospitable kitchen, where, after a supper of Exmouth sprats, they went to bed, while we talked birds to our hearts' content.

At the time of writing (December 1968) two of the birds taken to Exmouth are still alive, Janni and Bulgy. The Mini-guillie's fate has already been mentioned; a fate she might have met with in her natural surroundings. Poor Mr. Kwak spent a few more happy months, with expert attention to his feet, but we never really expected him to live long. Finally he developed the cough which is the symptom of the dreaded aspergillosis, for which there is no known cure. Mrs. Marsault went to infinite trouble to get a new apparatus similar to that used for asthma patients, but it was of no avail. Janni has so far remained healthy, inseparable from Bulgy who, alas, has recently developed a curious lack of balance, which seems to indicate something akin to a stroke or some other injury to the brain.

The inevitable question crops up. Is it worth it? Would it not be better to destroy these birds? This is something only the individual can answer for himself, for it is a question of his philosophy of life, of his attitude to the Schweitzerian 'reverence for life'. 'He who does not value life, does not deserve it,' wrote Leonardo da Vinci, five centuries ago,* and I would like to think he meant not only one's own life but life in all its forms, the forms he was so passionately absorbed in realising and interpreting in his art.

To the question 'Is it worth it?' there can be, for myself, only one answer. 'Yes' a thousand times 'Yes'; but not to prolong suffering. If a bird is clearly in incurable pain then let a whiff of chloroform or a Veterinary Surgeon's injection put it to sleep as gently as possible. But if there is a shred, only a shred of hope, or if the bird clings to life, then the battle must be fought to the end. Thoughts and feelings are not only sources of action but are a different sort of action in themselves, as every hermit or 'holy man' understands, and every action, thought or feeling which genuinely expresses a reverence for suffering life and, therefore, an acceptance of a portion of the burden of responsibility for that suffering, contributes in some indefinable measure to the sum total of positive or constructive forces in the affairs of man in his precarious relationship to the universe.

This is not a sentimentality; it is a declaration of faith.

Winter Postscript (27th December, 1968).

Since writing the above, the wreck of the Norwegian tanker, the *Sitakund*, has come to rest off our coast and there has been more oil in the channel. I have recently had two guillemot

* *The Notebooks of Leonardo da Vinci* (arranged by Edward MacCurdy Volume I) published by The Reprint Society.

patients. The first one, which was a strong handsome bird came in on 18th December and died on Friday, 20th December. The post mortem revealed highly inflamed intestines with apparently imminent ulceration. Even after two days in ice-cold water the guts stank of oil. Nothing, so far as one knows, could have saved it. It died peacefully, just after I had put it down from my lap.

The second one arrived the day the other one died, on Friday, 20th December and died during the night of 25th-26th December. As soon as it arrived it gratefully snuggled up to the warmth (Dimplex radiator and hot-water bottles) but was not interested either in food or water. (The first one had drunk fresh water from a cup.) It continued to do no more than give a desultory peck at a sprat, but after the first day, it never speared and swallowed one. It also slept almost continuously. I force-fed it, but it grew weaker. On Christmas Day I fed it small bits of fish every hour. During the whole of the week it sometimes regurgitated the hand-fed fish. It did not excrete as abundantly as guillemots do, and what it ejected was not black oil, but an evil-smelling mustard-yellow liquid. Both these guillemots, a short while before death, took up the unusual position of lying down with wings half-extended, as though to try and take some of the weight off the abdomen, and laid their heads forward on the ground. When they died, quietly, the head fell to one side.

At least they did not die, helpless, in the freezing cold, on a storm-blown beach, but unterrified, in warmth and quiet with food beside them. I used to visit them several times a night, and they would lift their heads with a momentary bright look, then sink back into sleep against the warmth.

One must ever keep in mind what Dorothy Yglesias wrote in her inspiring book.* 'It must be remembered that wild birds only allow themselves to be caught when their condition is pretty desperate; therefore, the number of complete cures is bound to be relatively small and the number of deaths great.' The death of a gentle guillemot is infinitely sad.

* *The Cry of a Bird* by Dorothy Yglesias. Published William Kimber 1962.

'Comment on doit quitter la vie et tous ses maux,
C'est vous qui le savez, sublimes animaux!'

says Alfred de Vigny in *La Mort du Loup*, and at the silence of their suffering, one enters into that stern poet's feelings.

Largely as a result of the oiled sea-birds problem there has been a tendency to think of centralising bird-help. Centralisation, as a principle, inevitably rouses feelings of concern in those who have experienced its less happy results in the educational field, for example. That the concentration of power or influence rarely has edifying effects on the wielders of it and is thus far from benevolent in its results has been repeatedly and tragically demonstrated in the history of human affairs. To suppose that when applied to creatures as utterly defenceless as sick birds, such measures would prove any less open to abuse is surely nothing more than a sentimental evasion of reality. De-centralisation into small 'cells' of amateur help, linked by the same aims and principles and working co-operatively, pooling and exchanging the knowledge gained from practical experience is infinitely sounder and safer because certainly less exposed to abuse. It is true one can never eliminate a margin of error but one can at least narrow it down. One is continually coming across little pockets of bird-help created by wholly devoted and disinterested people, seeking neither publicity nor power, who are doing splendid work, and here I am sure the hope for the future lies.

CHAPTER NINE

Binkie the Gallant

Whenever I think of Binkie, the adjective 'gallant' swims up alongside his image in the way that such adjectives do in the advertisements on the cinema screen. And what a strange little image it is.

'Looks more and more like a starling,' the V.S. said disparagingly, with affection in his voice.

Binkie is a cock blackbird; at least that is only rather dubiously established. After his first moult, he emerged feathered black, but at the time of writing (January 1969) his beak is not yellow, so in default of information, we assume that it will go yellow later.*

Binkie must have been born towards the end of June 1968, and he arrived at College at the beginning of July. It was a late fledgeling season that year. Most birds, after a catastrophic and early start seemed to have struggled with a second family. I had another blackbird fledgeling, uninjured, but a stray which the Veterinary Surgeon's wife had rescued and brought to me. As he was in perfect health and acted as if he were, he was called 'Frisky'. I was suffering from a mild degree of bathroom crowding so he had to share a cage with a fledgeling thrush whose parents had either deserted him or met with disaster themselves. He was about the same age as the blackbird, and they got on very well; in fact I witnessed an extraordinary thing. Frisky actually *fed* Thrushy. The first time this was clearly an accident. I used to feed them both with eyebrow-tweezers and Frisky had opened his beak and received a worm. He had not swallowed it and it dangled moustache-wise in his beak. Thrushy turned towards Frisky with beak wide open and speedily the worm was deposited in Thrushy's

* April 1969. Binkie's beak is now yellow.

beak. He lost no time in swallowing it. I decided this was an amusing accident. The second time that it happened it was no accident. I have my records before me. Frisky bent forward and deliberately placed his beakful in Thrushy's open beak. This happened altogether three or four times. Both birds were very strong, uninjured and both were released from the open-air aviary. Both still meet me from time to time in the Park. Thrushy returned to the aviary on several occasions, to look for titbits—and got them.

Into this bathroom fledgeling hurly-burly came Binkie. He had a wing-injury beyond repair with bone sticking out. He must have been hit or crushed by something. He could not stand. I gave the usual treatment for shock; a drink of glucose water, then on to a warm nest on a small hot-water bottle at the bottom of my cat-basket, which I placed on a box, level with a wall Dimplex radiator, the lid of the basket leaning against the radiator. I was thus enabled to drape a towel from the lid over one half of the basket to give Binkie a sheltered feeling. At the same time it was at a convenient level for feeding without having to move anything. The cage with the other fledgelings was nearby, and Binkie seemed to register their cheerful chirpings.

There seemed very little reason why Binkie should live, he was so small, so squashed, with the remains of one wing hanging down; and yet if ever there was a manifestation of the Schweitzerian 'will-to-live' it resided in this gallant scrap of feathers. Binkie ate with gusto; hard-boiled yolk of egg; brown granary bread soaked in diluted gold-top milk, sultanas, garden worms, meal-worms, shreds of lamb, bits of apple and cheese, and, as a special treat, ripe raspberries. As he could not move, and in spite of valiant efforts to excrete over the edge of his blanket 'nest' he had to be lifted fairly frequently during the day. I soon lined the blanket hollow with a fresh Kleenex tissue each time it got soiled, a simple and practical arrangement causing the bird the minimum of discomfort.

Dorothy Yglesias had once remarked 'Wherever you *first* make your bird comfortable and whatever you do *first*, that's what you'll have to stick to, because the bird will never accept, or be happy with, anything else.' I had many times experienced confirmation of this observation, but as I daily washed out Binkie's bijoux blankets, I could not help reflecting how much this applied to human beings too; at least it did in my own case. Ever since my first childhood experiences with birds, I have never been able to bring myself to place sick or young birds on anything but soft warm material; never, of course, on anything thready or with a frayed edge because the bird's feet, beak or neck could become fatally entangled. I have found hay or straw most unsatisfactory. The droppings get congealed in it; the bird gets wet and sticky and entangled; the food gets lost in it and mixed up with the droppings. I stick to blankets, and was interested to read in Joan Hicks' book that she, too, found them the most satisfactory thing.

Binkie throve, but suddenly I noticed an appalling smell. I had washed the wound with an antiseptic, but there was no mistaking the smell. It was gangrene. Horror-struck I telephoned the Veterinary Surgeon who told me to take Binkie to the surgery immediately. I rushed him down in his basket.

'I'll have to take this bone out,' said the Veterinary Surgeon. 'But the gangrene's not deep; I'll give him a special deep penicillin injection.' Then he added, 'He wants to live doesn't he?'

Gratefully, I assented.

The operation was performed, and I watched the hypodermic syringe as the V.S. skilfully injected the healing serum. Binkie stood up to it all with unwinking eye. I had brought three raspberries with me, and as soon as he was replaced in the basket, I produced them. He ate all three, much to the amusement of the Veterinary Surgeon and his assistants. I was given a tube of penicillin to treat the wound at regular intervals during the day.

Thankfully I returned to College. I did not care to contemplate what I would have felt if there had been any suggestion of putting Binkie to sleep. There had been no such suggestion; only encouragement. Now it was up to the nursing. The penicillin made Binkie very wet and coldish down one side. I pepped up his hot-water bottles, and pounded a third of a Binerva multi-vitamin tablet and mashed it into a little butter on a crumb of bread. I repeated this dose daily for about a fortnight. I continued to give glucose water which he took eagerly from a very small teaspoon.

After three days he went back to the surgery for another examination. The danger was over; the flesh was clean, but another bit of bone had to be removed. Thereafter Binkie's progress was smooth and steady. His feathers grew and eventually one day he tottered on to a leg, holding up the one on the injured side. His appetite never failed throughout all his trials, and he greeted my appearance with vociferous and enthusiastic anticipation. He settled down to his sleep regularly at night, and whenever I visited him to make sure all was well he never exhibited any signs of restlessness or discomfort. While he was so very ill I always replenished his hot-water bottle during the night, and this attention was appreciated. He would sink down against the fresh heat with engaging gladness.

Up to this point he had never left his basket. Now that he was slightly more active, I flattened the blanket over the floor of the basket, and arranged a 'nest bit' by piling up the material at one end. Binkie now took a shaky little step or two on the bottom of the basket but mostly he still reposed in or leaning against his nest. One day I asked one of my teachers if she would care to see Binkie. She gazed down on the small brown head lifted enquiringly in the basket. 'Yes, that's all very well, Mrs. Engholm,' she said severely, 'but what sort of a *future* has it got?'

At this point Binkie, much concerned with the present, gave a tweet, and joyfully received a mealworm on a snippet of Caerphilly, which he preferred to Cheddar (though what he really liked was Danish Blue).

'What sort of a future has it got?' This, naturally, had been the question in the forefront of my mind, ever since I had taken over his crushed little body. I had had to face at once, that if he lived he would remain a permanent resident. This entails a responsibility different from that involved in restoring birds which will be released, and one which should not be undertaken lightly. For one thing it constitutes a permanent tie. There is the question of holidays, for instance. One can find someone reliable to look after healthy pigeons without feeling guilty about it, but a crippled blackbird requiring a special diet, attention and exercise, is another matter. But from the first moment Binkie's 'will-to-live' shone brightly in his eyes. No human being worthy of the adjective could have resisted the silent appeal. I banished from my mind visions of a 1969 ski-ing holiday and accepted the responsibility with all its implications.

Now, as I write, six months later, I ask myself if anyone else in England has a blackbird to serenade them in the bath, for Binkie invariably celebrates the combination of company and the sound of bath-water! There is also the bird's side of it to be considered. Is its life in the crippled state going to be worth living? In Binkie's case he would not have to adjust from the wild, untrammelled state to a restricted one, since I had had him from fledgeling-hood, and he had known no other environment. Nevertheless his needs and demands as an adult would be more complex and there was the question of companionship, and possibly a wife. I thought it likely that some other blackbird victim would turn up and that in due course he might be granted a female friend. I had seen Rider and Hedger, the two venerable gulls which Dorothy Yglesias and her sister had rescued after they had each had a wing cut off by the wire of the practice-target towed by the Air Force 'planes. They lived a contented Darby and Joan existence in dignified serenity. I hoped I might achieve a similar solution for Binkie and took the risk.

Since writing the above, I did, in fact, one evening receive an injured female blackbird, and feeling much as one does when stuffing a child's Christmas stocking, I placed her in Binkie's pen. Binkie became very excited and made soft, tender noises. Within half an hour the newcomer had booted (literally in this case) Binkie from his nightly shoe-roost which she had immediately appropriated, while Binkie huddled in cowed submission on the box below. I erected another shoe on the rack and helped Binkie on to it. He spent a hen-pecked night while the aggressive visitor enjoyed his draught-proof perch and next day I removed the untamed shrew to another site whereupon

Binkie revived and carolled his relief at returning to normal bachelordom.

When we had finally finished off our July and August summer holiday courses, I decided to snatch a fortnight's respite at my cottage, before plunging once more into what promised to be a more than usually demanding Christmas term. The usual stresses and strains of the past months had been acerbated by the unconstructive antics of catering firms, (what a gold-mine for the cartoonist!) and I longed to be boiling my own free range egg in the calm and uncontended precincts of my tiny kitchen, with its floor of rich purply brick. By this time Binkie was lop-sidedly mobile and I had to work out a safe modus vivendi for him, within his new environment. Accordingly I fixed his wire-fronted 'cage'—with its door propped open—on a box level with the kitchen table, and placed his scratching tray of earth in front of it.

My kitchen table is good solid stuff, probably home-made, with a marvellously functional drawer. I had discovered it in the basement of a junk-shop and—much to the shop-owner's chagrin—with an unambiguous price label still attached. With foxy cunning he had detected the gleam in my eye which betrayed that more might have been wrung out of me. I plonked down the cash while he was still muttering, and with a hastily-constructed cardboard number plate flapping from my new acquisition had managed to reach the last roundabout in Seaside before being gonged by the police. Distracted I pointed out that there was no delivery of furniture to my rural residence. The officers were kindly and helpfully suggested they would stuff the thing into the car for me. Knowing this to be an impossibility I aided the operation which terminated with the table on the pavement and much head-scratching. Finally the whole thing was tied up again as before and after warning me not to exceed 30 m.p.h. I set off without further frustration for I have never in my life cherished ambitions concerning the speed limit.

Now the commodious top of this imposing piece, provided play-pen room for Binkie, while allowing me to enjoy my meals alongside. Binkie was enthralled and used to whip the bacon-rind off my plate, charging off importantly to wipe it in the earth before disposing of it in stages.

The table was too high for him to venture a jump; he was realising his limitations, but after breakfast I used to lift him on to the floor. If it was a sunny morning the back door opposite the table would be open, and after bathing in the dog's drinking water, he would hop on to the wooden bar at the bottom of the doorway, and preen. At such moments he looked appalling; more like the animated head of a dish-mop or as I felt I would look if luckily regurgitated by a whale; a sorry advertisement indeed for my bird-care. On a dull day he went straight to the small electric heater and dried off in front of that, often spreading out a fan-like wing, as blackbirds do in the sun.

Everything about cottage life delighted Binkie. No bird was ever more at home. I felt a telepathic chord of sympathy between his frail bird-spirit and my clumsy human one—and I respected his efforts to establish an increasing independence. I kept a diary of his doings, and a typical day went something like this:

BINKIE'S DAY

6.30 a.m. I would come down to make my morning tea, and would look to see what Binkie had eaten off the saucer I left beside his scratching tray when I went up to bed at night. It was a mixture of cheese, hard-boiled egg, blackberries, or elderberries and a few brown bread-crumbs. Usually he had polished off most of it and I would give him his first morning feed while my kettle boiled. Having been hand-reared he still liked the attention of being hand-fed, though by this time completely capable of self-feeding. I would then leave him to scratch around on his tray while I had my tea in bed, wrote letters or read.

8 a.m.-ish. I came down and if the weather was fine (by that I mean not utterly impossible!) I would work in the garden. First I would give Binkie another snack, then I would lift him from the table and put him on the kitchen floor and leave the back door open. Binkie adored this bit of the day and so did I.

While I gardened I could keep an eye on Binkie. He did not, at first, venture far from the back door. I had put down broken paving stones outside my back door in an amateurish crazy paving. Binkie would peer down the cracks and pick out little bits of gravel. He ate a good deal of what appeared to be 'pure' earth as well as grit, but apart from what he swallowed he greatly enjoyed scratching in the gravelly soil under the wooden garden seat outside the back door, hurling broken bits of brick about and carrying around stones of considerable size. I weighed one once and it weighed over half an ounce. Once a stone he had dislodged hit the dustbin with a ping; this startled him and he stiffened, but not for long.

One morning he carried round and bullied a piece of bacon-rind for a solid hour, and then to my astonishment he dropped it and craned over backwards till he nearly lost his balance to look up at an aeroplane passing overhead. He relaxed when it had gone over, scratched, retrieved his bacon-rind and ate it on a stone. At the time I doubted whether I had interpreted his behaviour correctly, but as at every subsequent appearance of an aeroplane in the sky, he gave a swift look upwards and then shot into the kitchen, there could be no mistaking the connection. I have noted in my diary that he was always (and he still is) acutely conscious of things in the sky or above him. I presume that owing to his physical handicap a descent from the sky in the shape of another blackbird, for example, would spell danger for him in a way that would not effect a non-handicapped bird.

10.30 a.m.-ish. I usually stopped gardening and had breakfast at the kitchen table. If sunny, the back door remained open and Binkie either rested on the doorstep or somewhere in a patch of sunlight in the kitchen. If he was very come-hitherish I put him on the table and he shared bits off my plate. I had to be careful not to hurt my collie's feelings, so he used to sit or lie beside my chair, not for bits, as he was the ungreediest of dogs, but for the sake of feeling included.

After a leisurely breakfast I sometimes had a bath. My bath is the smallest size available and I had it installed in the place of the old copper, leaving as much of the old brickwork as possible, which prompted the Duke of Devonshire's agent to remark to his architect through whose kind auspices the installation had taken place, 'I hear you've put a bath in a chimney now!' Bathing, therefore, has for me—and for most of my guests—a special charm. Village callers, such as the baker, who makes oven-baked bread, quickly summed up its position and my daily rhythm, so that they would whistle loudly as they rounded the rainwater butt and then halt diplomatically by the garden seat. Thus suitably warned I could either emerge, or else shout 'one small cob, please' or whatever instructions were required. One of the everlasting joys of cottage life is the ever-open back door and the feeling this engenders of being on a never-ending and luxurious camping holiday, in constant contact with the earth but without the earwigs in the pillow. After my bath, I usually went to do my shopping at the village shop, which meant shutting Binkie into the kitchen. If he seemed sleepy or inactive I put him on the table and he then frequently retired into his cage. He could not perch so I had put a thick piece of branch on the cage floor—like a junior log—and it formed his favourite seat. If, on the other hand, he exhibited signs of being spry, I left him on the floor where he always found something to amuse him, pulling paper bags out of the dust-pan, and stirring up the contents of the ground floor shelf under the draining-board beside the sink, thus painfully exposing to the public eye my unhousewifely cupboard failings. He rapidly eliminated spiders, and stray woodlice, and would launch himself into the void in pursuit of a bluebottle or a moth. In fact, he exhibited all the characteristic blackbird 'busy-ness' alternating with periods of immobility or rest. Before leaving him I used to put down his saucer of bits.

On my return and depending on the weather he usually came into the garden again; I would read or I would continue to garden and he would spread himself in the sun to sunbathe. He also discovered that by means of a series of 'wing-hops' he could scale the manure heap next to the dustbin and this provided him with endless occupation.

3-4 p.m.-ish. After a cup of tea, I again shut Binkie into the kitchen while I took the dog for a walk. Sometimes I drove over to College to deal with some correspondence and was away for two or three hours.

6 p.m.-ish. The evenings were as softly relaxed as the mornings. Binkie was ready for his supper and then settled himself for the night. As I always go to bed very early at the cottage, I would give him a last raspberry or mealworm before turning out the light and making my way up the few stairs that separate my first from my ground floor.

And so the days passed peacefully in a tranquil country rhythm, punctuated by unexpected Binkie variations. For instance, one morning while drinking my tea in bed, I heard curious noises below. As the floorboards of the cottage are ancient and full of cracks, no one, not even a bird, could lead a secret life within its walls. I assumed that Binkie was having a particularly happy scratch on his tray and paid no more attention; though there was an odd kind of rhythm about the noise. Later when I was about to descend the stairs—which are dark—I saw a dark lump on the stair beneath the top one. I thought I must have dropped a sock, but it moved and was—Binkie! With incredible effort he had hauled himself up seven of the eight stairs to my bedroom, but the last one—being deeper than the others—had defeated him. I rewarded him with many titbits. The self-same evening as I was drinking my after-supper coffee in bed, I heard the same noises. This time I got up and found Binkie on the bottom stair about to re-essay his ascent. I returned him to his bed and thenceforth shut the kitchen door—regretfully be it said, but it was in the interests of Binkie's safety.

At this time Binkie was still rather dependent on me. If, in the garden, he momentarily disappeared under a bush and I called him, he would always answer, and once when he was resting beside my clump of Dorsetshire pinks, I heard alarmed cries. I went out and found Binkie in a state; when I tried to pick him up he fled and cried piteously, but when eventually I did catch him he leant against me and calmed down. I took him indoors and put him on the kitchen table. He at once took refuge in the farthest corner of his cage and although it was only 3 p.m. he did not come out again that day. I never

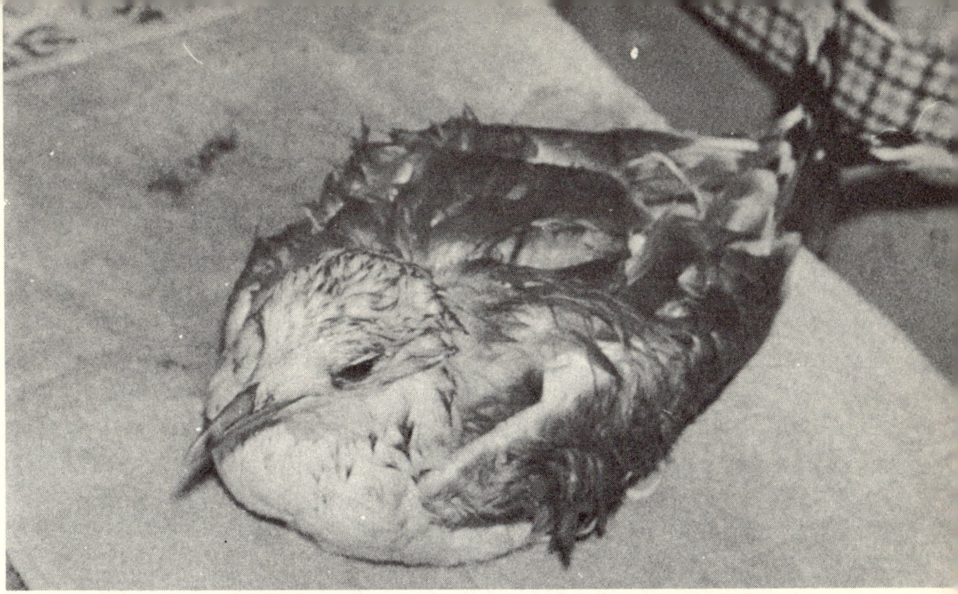

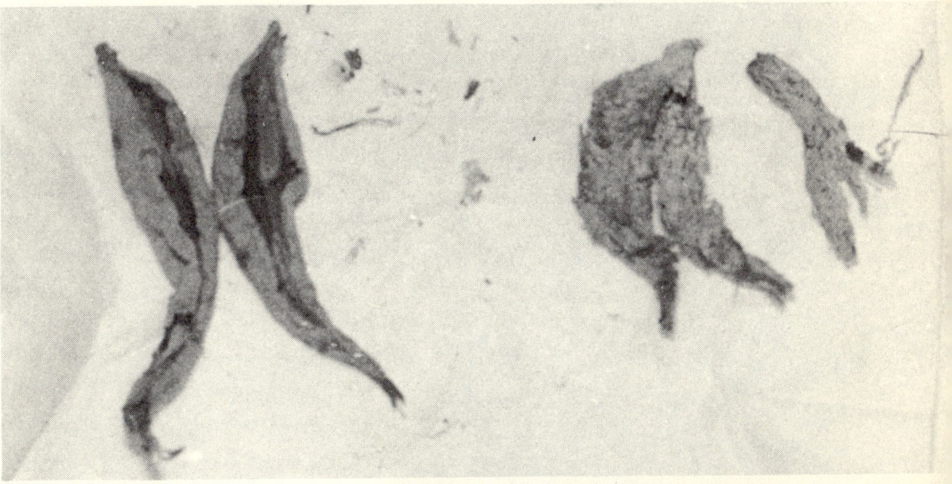

(Top). Gull (Belinda)—found on beach non-waterproof.

(Centre). Dahlia tuber, cut longitudinally on left. Belinda's vomited dahlia tuber on right (shrunk after an interval of 3 days).

(Right). Belinda in outside aviary feeling better after having got rid of her tuber!

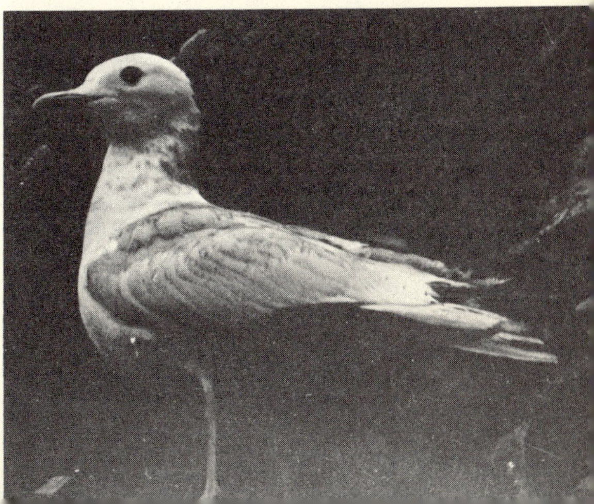

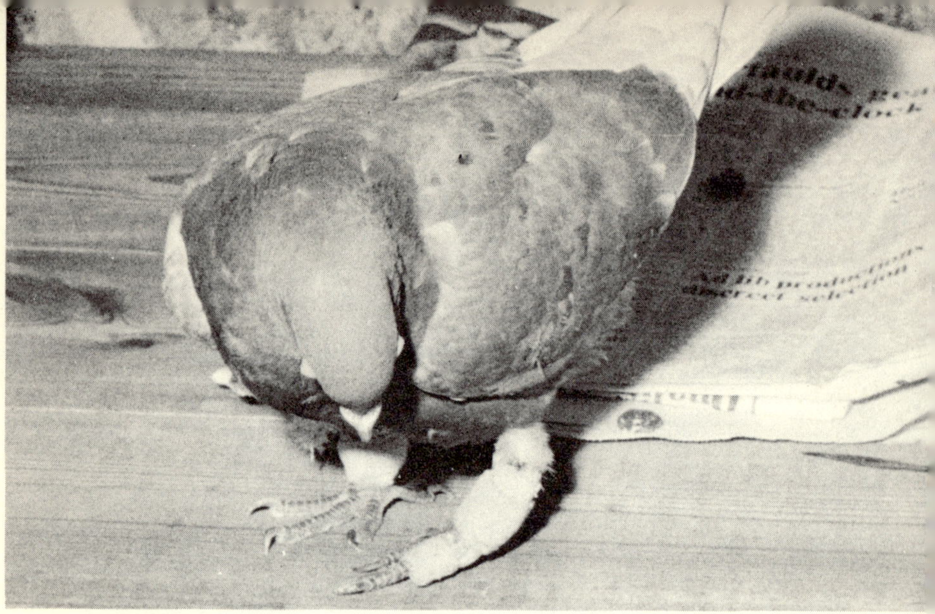

Mrs. Bates, in splints after she could stand. Note bent leg which was the leg with a double fracture.

Mrs. Bates at half-time. Much improved in health and some of the dressing removed.

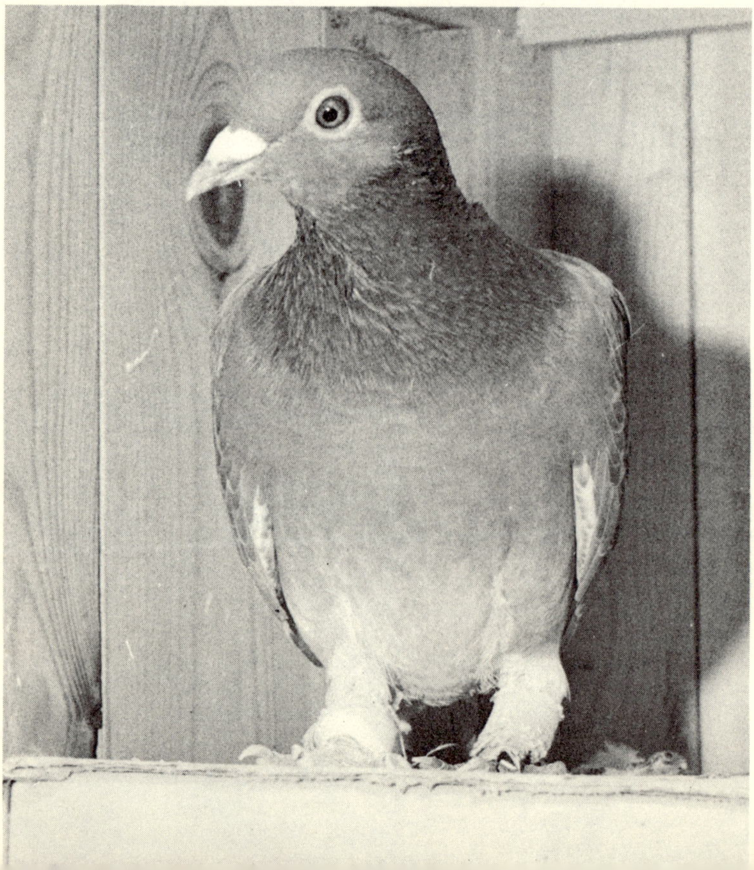

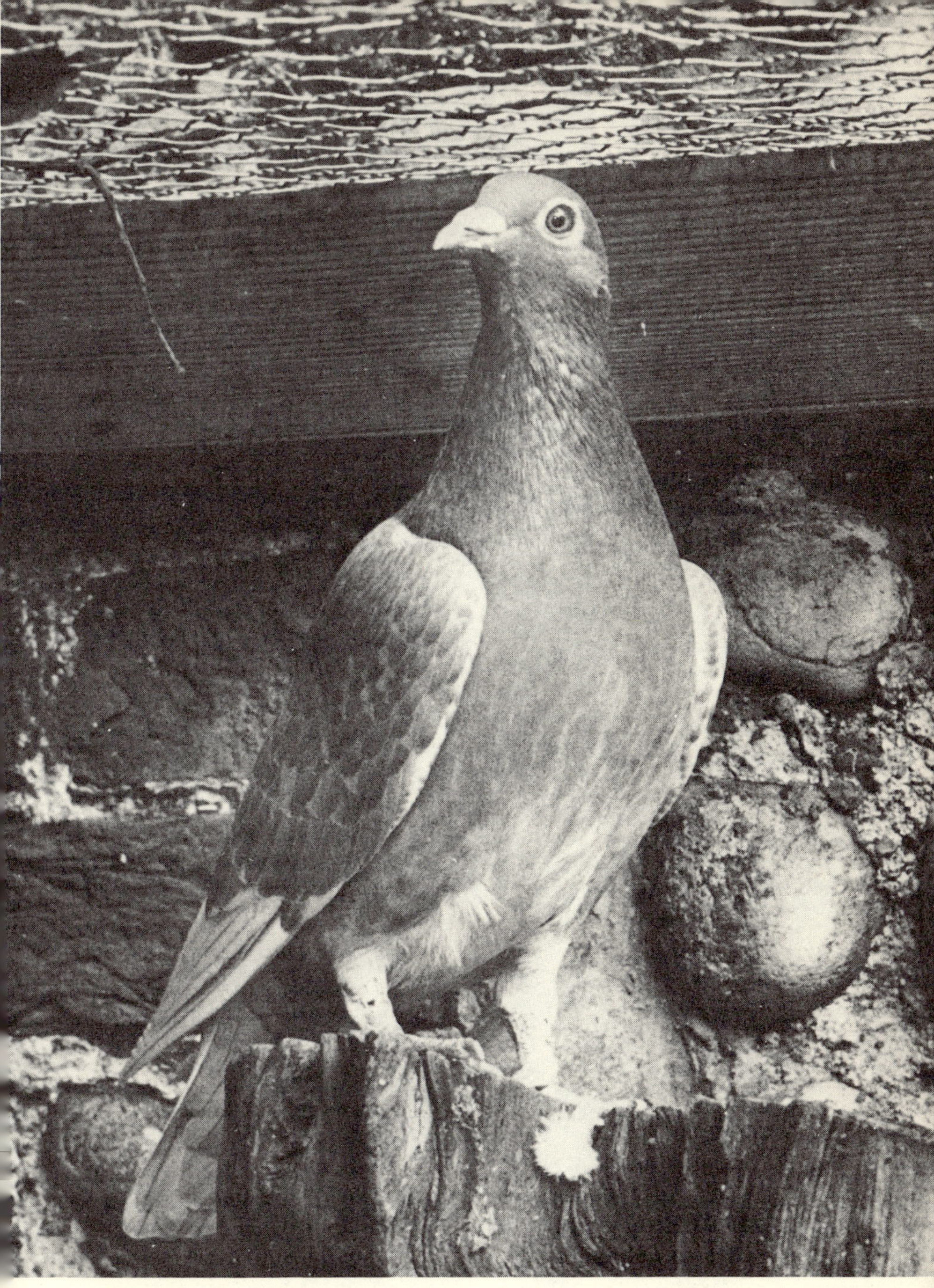

Mrs. Bates, in outside pen, with splints off. She is now flying free.

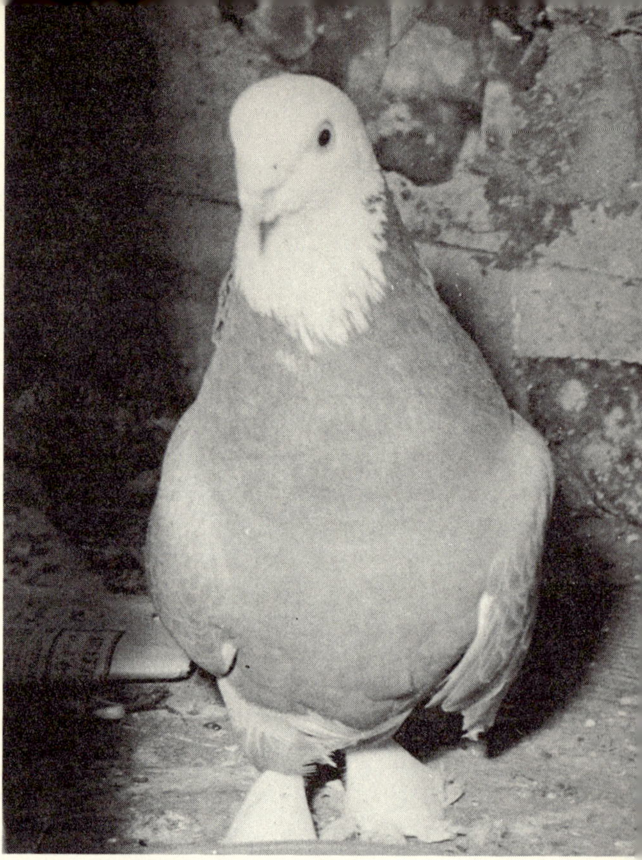

Trousers Ming, our pigeon receptionist. 'And what can I do for you Modom?'

'Would you care to see your room?'

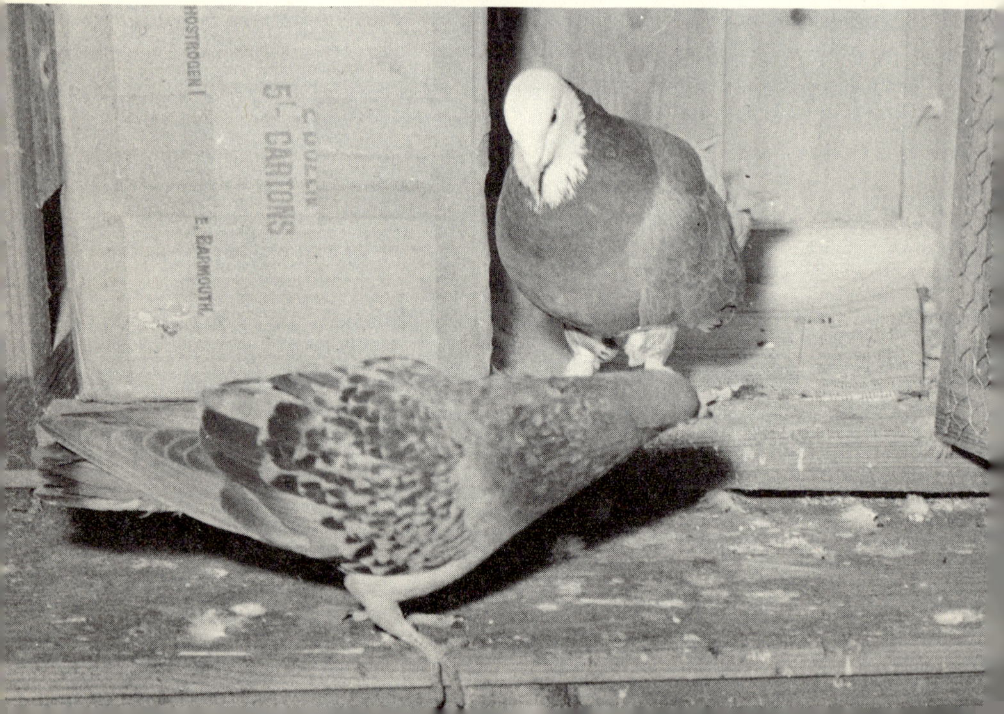

discovered the cause of his fright; my neighbours had no cats at this time, but I think that possibly another cock blackbird may have attacked him.

On rainy days Binkie adored bathing in the puddles, especially the one on the lid of the drain by the back door. After getting thoroughly sodden, Binkie—with many self-congratulatory flicks—would make his way to the electric heater to get dry. If I had not turned it on I would see him spread out in front of it—an irresistible appeal.

One afternoon I suddenly realised he had not come in and it was pouring outside. I could not see him in his favourite spots and was just beginning to feel anxious when suddenly from beneath the dripping wooden seat beside the door there issued forth a soft little chuckling song, such as an Irish 'fairy' might have sung. It was Binkie's first venture into the musical field.

Binkie began to moult and I began to worry. He went distinctly bald on top, and very scraggy about the neck. He also developed a brilliant yellow ring round each eye. Other feathers dropped out, including his tail feathers. He maintained his vitality, appetite and general good spirits, while I took stock of every blackbird that crossed my path. Previously, of course, I had noticed blackbirds in a similar state on the bird-table, but I simply could not decide if the symptoms were normal or presaging some disease or dietary deficiency. I rang up Dorothy Yglesias whose first question was an enquiry as to Binkie's general health and behaviour. When I told her this did not seem to be affected she reassured me by advising me, in this case, to leave well alone; it was probably just a very bad moult, and considering Binkie's difficult fledgeling-hood, not altogether surprising.

By the time I returned to College at the end of September, he looked a mess but was beginning to change colour, growing visibly darker. Finally, to my great relief, he became entirely re-feathered—in black—and the bright yellow eye-rings took on a gentler hue. Nevertheless, even now—February 1969—Binkie presents an unfinished appearance, for no tail has been provided, as though somehow the supply of feathers had run out. He ends in a frayed edge, reminiscent of Victorian mantelpiece fringes. I entertain great hopes of this deplorable omission being repaired during his next moult. What the yellow rims round the eye denote I do not know. Some cock blackbirds have them; others, and, in my limited experience these seem to be in the majority, have not. I have given up worrying, as Binkie continues to flourish.

Back at College, I established Binkie in the smaller aviary outside, bringing him in at night to the bathroom. To my surprise he moped, so I left the door open and allowed him out into the larger aviary. I knew he could not get out, but it was frequently visited by other blackbirds and Binkie's fright at the cottage lingered in my mind. However, he clearly enjoyed the larger aviary which was full of old rotten logs and leaf-mould, and where he found numbers of slugs, his favourite natural food. Binkie never much cared for worms (except meal-worms!) but he was a gourmand as far as slugs were concerned. I was intrigued by this, as in my experience birds generally found slugs too slimy and avoided them. Not Binkie; he had a special technique. He would wipe the slug back and forth in the earth, and he did this until the slug was reduced to a kind of worm with not a vestige of anything slimy about it. Then when at its most earthy, he would swallow it with obvious satisfaction.

Occasionally he would apply this technique to an ordinary earthworm, but he generally abandoned the worm in the end. He searched for slugs by indefatigably turning over leaves; I rather think that this is also what the blackbirds in the Park are doing when they are busy among the undergrowth. True, they pick up other insects too, but the chief aim would appear to be slugs. Binkie did not confine himself to dead leaves; he used to examine all my primulas, and de-slug them most efficiently. Unlike thrushes he had no use for snails, except the very small variety, mostly to be found under rotten wood.

Binkie was becoming fiercely independent, and round about this time he gave up answering to my call. This constituted a problem for me as it sometimes took me some time to locate him in the large aviary. A very handsome adult cock with orange beak and rapacious intentions used to arrive as soon as I put down food for Binkie. While I remained in the aviary I could keep order but I suspected that a certain amount of aggression went on when I was not there. Binkie was quick to realise that his only defence was to dive underneath protective covering; hence I used to find him under the logs in little hollows, apparently calm and unruffled, but the evening when I had to dismantle almost the entire log-pile, to find him, I decided that it was time I invented a better programme. Actually it was getting colder, and Binkie felt the cold. I had observed in Woolworth's one of the old-fashioned fireguards, of the kind that used to be placed around nursery fires. I went to investigate. This resulted in one of those mysterious shopping dramas which seem to dog my innocent footsteps. I was delighted to see the required article, still safely on its shelf. Pointing to it I asked a reluctant assistant if I might have it.

'Wot? That?'

'Yes, please.'

'That fireguard?'

'Yes, that's right; the fireguard.'

She gave me a swift and hostile look, and promptly vanished in the crowd. Baffled, I was turning to seek another assistant, when the plastic paraphernalia lady caught my eye and said with would-be helpfulness 'Gone downstairs.' From this I concluded that rather than ascend some steps to haul down the guard on the shelf, the assistant had descended into the Woolworthian bowels to haul another up. Five minutes passed, then ten and I grew restive. Observed by the compassionate plastics assistant, the latter called over the second of the lamp-shades assistants and asked her to stand by the plastics while she also descended into the cellar. Five more minutes went by, and then —oh triumph!—she reappeared dragging an enormous flat cardboard box. As the thing cost several pounds, and in spite of the picture on the box, I asked if I could get it out in order to see if 'it worked', i.e. that once out of its collapsed state, it would stand up without wobbling, and that all the hooks and eyes fitted. Great was the ensuing consternation. We were joined by an elderly Yorkshire woman who with Northern sense and thriftiness correctly appraised the situation, and I won my point. Finally at the end of forty minutes I staggered out with Binkie's new play-pen.

I erected the pen at the 'guillemot' end of the bathroom, that is to say by the low Dimplex radiator, and put the cage Binkie had had at the cottage at one end. Then I arranged a few logs in tiers so that Binkie could run up to the roof of his cage which was just below the top of my shoe-rack. Binkie thoroughly approved of this arrangement, and thereafter roosted nightly on one of my shoes. To begin with, I still took him to the outside aviary (the smaller one) for a few hours every day, but he so obviously preferred the bathroom pen, that I soon gave up.

Binkie now resented being handled; indeed I had always handled him as little as possible in deference to his natural desire for independence. Now he would snap at me with sharp clicks of his beak, but would consent to be carried if allowed to perch of his own accord on my hand. 'Perch' is not really a very good word to describe his stance, as he had not much grip in his feet, and preferred flat surfaces, so that he clung to two or three fingers at a time or else stood in my hand or on my arm. He was quite happy like that, but any suggestion of restriction such as cupping one's hands around him, he felt to be humiliating and fought back.

Whenever I had a 'free' afternoon I drove over to my cottage to do some gardening, and I used to take Binkie with me in the cat-basket.

The first time I returned to the cottage with Binkie after our holiday there I was wondering whether he would remember anything, but I never imagined to what extent he would resume his cottage habits. As soon as we arrived, I fetched the key from the toolshed and opened the back door; then putting the basket down just outside it, I lifted the lid and tilted the basket so that Binkie could get out. He hopped out, looked around, went straight into the kitchen, turned right and immediately splashed into the dog's bowl to bath as usual. I turned on the heater, and from then on he picked up his cottage 'pattern'. He had, however, become an adult, and he was far more venturesome than before. I was, therefore, compelled to build a rough pen extending from the back door, to ensure his safety. Inside the pen was a little covered wire 'run' originally used to protect a short row of lettuces. If ever Binkie felt slightly insecure he rushed into this little run, but if he really felt threatened, he dashed into the kitchen and hid under the duster box beside the bath. After this visit I nearly always took him with me. It had been a splendid blackberry season, and somewhere along a hedge on the drive back to College I used to pick a handful of blackberries, and as we drove along I occasionally popped one into the basket. This was greeted by an appreciative 'chuck, chuck!' and by the time we got to College there were never any berries left.

The autumn wore on and at the end of October I got my first new season's guillemot, presumed victim of the escaping sludge oil from the Norwegian tanker, the *Sitakund*, which had caught fire and run aground off Eastbourne beach. We called this guillemot 'Sita', and as Matron pointed out he *was* our seventh guillemot and 'Sita' is the word for seven in Swahili. (Matron had done her stint in Africa too.)

I was thankful for such experience as I had had with guillemots, for at least I was now familiar with 'the drill', and had my special box of medical impedimenta for guillemots.

As Binkie was now occupying the Woolworth's play-pen at one end of the bathroom I made another little snug place for Sita at the other end. Later on I noticed Sita seemed rather restless and averse to being 'captive'. I thought I would try something and having spread a towel over a sponge-rubber square in front of Binkie's Dimplex (greatly to his interest) I placed Sita upon it. Binkie was on his log near the floor, about a foot and a half away. As soon as Sita had spotted Binkie, he spread his wings and advanced upon him as though to embrace him. He collapsed when he reached the log, while Binkie with a squawk of alarm retired to his shoe upon the shoe-rack. Sita got as close as possible to Binkie and then settled down contentedly, and exhibited no further signs of restlessness.

A most unlikely friendship immediately sprang up between these two ill-assorted birds. They seemed enchanted with each other, and Sita, in particular would not let Binkie out of his sight. He even tried to get into his cage, when Binkie was in it, though the door was much too small. As long as he was near Binkie Sita was content, and when Binkie ate, Sita would eat a little fish, so that we started to call Binkie 'Nurse Binkie'. On the day after Sita's arrival and while he was drying after his de-oiling, Binkie suddenly started to sing, and sang softly for about a quarter-of-an-hour. He had not done this since his effort in the rain at the cottage. Alas, the friendship was of brief duration. Sita was excreting jets of oil, and a couple of mornings later I heard Sita move a little at 6 a.m. and when I went to the bathroom to have a bath at 6.30 a.m. I found Sita apparently sitting quietly looking at Binkie. I did not turn on the light not wishing to disturb them, but when I had had my bath I thought I would feed Sita. He was still in exactly the same position which struck me as curious. I went across to him and saw that he was dead.

I removed the body hoping Binkie would not notice too much, but Binkie was inconsolable, moped, did not sing and pecked me with sharp snaps of his beak. I made great efforts to try and secure another guillemot but I did not get one till December. Then I had two, one after the other. The first was very ill and died almost at once; the second one seemed strong, stood well on its feet, and settled down very happily in Binkie's pen. Binkie was delighted, sang, flipped round the guillemot who watched him *almost*, one would have said, with tolerant amusement in his eye. This guillemot certainly did not respond in the way the first one had, but he was always friendly towards Binkie.

In spite of what might have been interpreted as initial progress I was very worried about the bird, and after five days he spent almost the whole of Christmas day on my lap and died that night.

Binkie was once more plunged into gloom, and it was at this point that Miss Raymonde-Hawkins so kindly presented me with Dorcas, the pigeon, and though she provided a distraction which helped Binkie over the loss of his guillemot, it was clear that Binkie would accept no substitutes.

At the time of writing—February 1969—Binkie has recovered his habitual cheerfulness and bounce. He has to be watched as he occasionally overshoots himself and loses his balance, thereby landing on his back. Sometimes he manages to right himself, but mostly he has to be helped on to his feet. He accepts these contretemps with his usual high-spirited gallantry, gives himself a good shake, looks at one mischievously, and sets off once more on his business. If I am out I always ask Matron if she will kindly visit him from time to time to make sure that he is all right.

Binkie is now in full voice. He has two sorts of vocal expression. One is a kind of soft, muted song, of full blackbird range, which he produces with his beak closed and often when he is cosily resting, with both feet tucked under him. The V.S. calls this his ventriloquist act! The other is a strong, positively piercing whistle, produced first thing in the morning and last thing at night with open beak.

One morning, while in my study, I was much taken aback to hear someone whistling for my dog. Slightly annoyed I went upstairs thinking it to be a student; there I found my Collie with a startled look and issuing from the bathroom and from Binkie, a faithful reproduction of my 'dog-whistle'. This has become one of Binkie's favourite whistles, and after a somewhat harassing apprenticeship my collie now ignores it, but only the other day some one exclaimed 'Who on earth is that whistling exactly like you for the dog?' When the reply is 'It's a blackbird in the bathroom', the questioner's credulity remains strained till the truth is demonstrated.

Other bird-patients continue to come and go in the bathroom, and though Binkie is interested, he is also jealous, and once the coast is clear again, the exodus is always celebrated by repeated bursts of song.

There is not much more to be said though every day with Binkie has its own unpredictable flavour.

But I think the last word on Binkie rests with Mrs. Rowland, the cleaner, who looking lovingly over the bathroom washbasin said 'That little bird; that's a *real* treasure!' (For Binkie's daily diet sheet see Appendix IV.)

CHAPTER TEN

A Chapter of Case-Histories

The case of Birling, the Blackbird

On 22nd July, the friend teaching immigrant children in London had arranged to take them for a day by the sea, and we were expecting them at College that afternoon to give us a short puppet performance, to meet some of our students of their nationality, and to drink unlimited Coca-Cola. In the middle of the morning, however, I received an S.O.S. from the teacher who was telephoning from the kiosk outside the Birling Gap Hotel to ask me to fetch a fledgeling blackbird. She rang off abruptly saying she feared some of the immigrants were drowning on the beach below. I drove over to Birling Gap immediately. Although the season was in full swing it was not difficult to locate her position from the polyglot cries arising from a multi-coloured scattering of children of a great variety of shapes and sizes. The one thing they seemed to possess in common was an overwhelming vitality. As I descended the steps the teacher caught sight of me and pointed to where she had deposited her belongings farther up the beach. We arrived at the spot simultaneously and she then explained that one of the Cypriots on his way to Victoria Station early that morning had been hailed by a motorist and ordered to pick up a fledgeling blackbird sitting in the middle of the road. He had obeyed and taken it with him to deliver it to his teacher at the station, knowing that she entertained quaint ideas on the subject of birds. The fledgeling was now huddled in her open and capacious handbag, over which she had hastily constructed some kind of awning. He looked frightened but robust and I transferred him into my cat-basket.

His rescuer was a warm-hearted lad who anxiously enquired after the fledgeling's welfare during his visit to the College that afternoon, and was much impressed on being shown 'Birling', as we had named him, fatly contented and happily established after a satisfying meal and duly enveloped in warm blankets.

Birling's progress while I was still at College was steady, but after the conclusion of the July course I was due to go to my cottage for a break. Birling came with me, together with one or two pigeons needing especial care. He settled down happily in the cottage kitchen, and as I had had to confine him for certain periods at College in a roomy cage, he had no objections to spending some of his time in this cage placed outside on the coal-bunker while I gardened or was otherwise busy. Suddenly he developed a cough. This 'coughing' greatly resembles 'sneezing' and sounds a little like 'tshew, tshew'! As the bird also shakes his head at the same time one is inclined to think it *is* sneezing and to dismiss it as something not very important. Experience had taught me otherwise. I watched Birling carefully. At first he did not cough often. About the third day, however, his coughing fits occurred more frequently and lasted longer. Having had him since he was a fledgeling I thought it unlikely that it was gapeworm. I decided that if I could use some harmless inhalant it might just possibly help. I always use Vapex when I have a cold myself so finally I took Birling on to my knee, soaked a blob of cotton-wool in Vapex and held it lightly over his nostrils. He was not at all put out; on the contrary he seemed to like it. I held the Vapexed cotton-wool to his nose for about one minute, and then took it away. To my surprise it worked like a charm. No more coughing or sneezing. I was greatly relieved.

Birling was now practically ready for his release. He had already spent a day or two in my fruit-cage (the wire-netting enclosure in which I grow raspberries and currants), to become more accustomed to scratching and picking up the food I put down. I still had to hand-feed him as well, of course. It is precisely this transitional stage which is so precarious and where one is so acutely conscious of one's human limitations. Unlike the mother-bird one is not able to follow the young bird on to a branch to feed it there, and yet, in spite of its picking up some food for itself (mostly actually found by its mother), it still needs to be fed. Gradually, but very gradually, the young bird finds more of its own food, and requires less feeding. The transition is never sudden. Hence I always dread these releases. They are the acid test. One false step in timing, or placing or method of releasing, and disaster follows.

I considered the pros and cons. Other blackbirds occupy my neighbours' gardens as well as appearing in my own to bath in the dustbin-lid kept full of water for that purpose. How would they re-act to a newcomer? One of the neighbours had acquired a cat, but it leads a persecuted existence in our area as I have trained my collie to overcome his infallible bonhomie towards all and sundry, sufficiently for him to bark and chase it. My next door neighbour, a bird lover also, throws her shoes at it; hence I hoped it would be kept at bay during the hazardous transition period before Birling became completely 'wild'. So much for the 'cons'.

On the 'pros' side, my kitchen door which is the back door, is always open so that Birling had constant and free access to it, if in danger or difficulty. There is a beautiful and prolific willow tree at the end of the garden, a safe harbour for many kinds of birds. Birling would have as good a chance as any.

On Thursday, 7th August, however, Birling took the initiative and flew from my lap out of the kitchen door. Next day he came back throughout the day to be fed. At first he perched on a branch above my compost heap where I could only just manage to reach him. Fortunately blackbirds tend to pursue, and as I moved away he fluttered after me. Thereafter he perched regularly on the coal-bunker (where I had left his cage with the door open), my wooden clothes horse or the bird-table, whenever he wanted to be hand-fed. One night we had a storm and a downpour of rain. I was interested to find Birling in his cage when I opened the back door in the morning. He was dry and ready for breakfast.

On 15th August, to my great alarm, I had him coughing in the hedge. Though he still fed occasionally from my hand, he no longer let me touch him and was generally independent.

I was much exercised as to how I would catch him to try and repeat the Vapex treatment. I worried all day, as I could hear him 'tschew, tschew-ing' in various parts of the garden. I did not get him that day but early next morning, when he came as usual for his breakfast of cheese on the coal-bunker, I was surprised to find that he let me pick him up. I took him indoors thinking hard. If I did not manage to scotch the cough properly and finally this time it was unlikely that Birling would let me handle him again. I asked myself what would I do on a desert island with a basic medicine chest and an emergency with a baby. I had in my medicine cupboard a bottle of Armstrong's Influenza Mixture which, recommended by my neighbour, had proved a godsend to me when submerged in an appalling 'fluey cold. After giving Birling the Vapex treatment as before, I made up my mind and gave him a few drops of the influenza mixture in a teaspoon. As it went down his eloquent eyes expressed surprise but not displeasure. He sat on my knee for a few moments 'taking it in', then with a flick he was off. Though I remained in touch with him a long time he never coughed again.

I told the Veterinary Surgeon who was very interested and examined the label on the Armstrong's Influenza Mixture bottle. It contained purely harmless ingredients of the so-called 'old-fashioned' kind. But it had done the trick, not only for me but for Birling.

The case of Birling, the blackbird, will live in my memory for two reasons. Firstly because he is the only bird I have ever cured of a cough and secondly because his release with its daily slackening of dependence went off so smoothly as to be perfect —and few things are ever that!

I always keep several receptacles full of clean water at my cottage and Birling still has his little bowl on the coal-bunker. (October 1969.)

The case of a nestful of House-Martins

At 9 a.m. on Friday, 5th September, the telephone rang. I was at my desk, ready to take morning Assembly. The voice of the Veterinary Surgeon said diffidently, 'I really hesitate to ask you ...' 'What is it?' I interrupted eagerly. 'Well, it's a nest of house-martins—three of them.' 'Right,' I said, 'I don't teach the first period after Assembly, I'll be round shortly.'

After Assembly I charged off to the surgery and the Veterinary Surgeon presented me with a minute box full of hay. Inside were two house-martins and a third one, so static that I said 'One's dead.' 'No, I don't think so,' said the Veterinary Surgeon. I touched it. It was still alive. 'Where have they come from?' I asked. 'An assistant in Boots found them on the ground, so she said. She'd taken them to a pet-shop but they wouldn't have them, so she brought them here.'

As soon as I got back, I gave the trio drops of glucose water. They seemed shocked but not cold. I put them inside my invaluable hairy hat in a basket next to the wall radiator in the bathroom. They still had bits of baby fluff adhering to their heads, so that the foreseeable length of stay merited supplying them with names. One of my favourite painters is Monet; one of my husband's used to be Manet. When staying in a crooked little hotel on the Ile de la Cité in Paris, my husband would sometimes suggest, 'Let's go and look at Minet, Manet and Monet today, shall we?' At that time I thought this would be the ideal nomenclature for a litter of kittens, but we never indulged in female cats. Now I thought it would do very well for the martins.

Minet and Manet stuck together, but Monet seemed rather apart. None of them opened their beaks and I had to force-feed them once every hour, resorting to the method employed for Speedy, the swift. I fed them bluebottles and tiny shreds of lamb. At 1 p.m. they started to twitter at the approach of food. At 6 p.m. that evening Manet—the middle one—opened his beak and clamoured. He ate 8-12 bits of lamb as well as flies before bedtime. At 6 a.m. next morning Minet—the littlest one—followed his example, but nothing would budge Monet. His beak resembled a pin and I nearly went demented levering it open with a fine hairpin, and then pushing in a fly or a bit of lamb with eyebrow-tweezers before withdrawing the hairpin. He ate with a certain degree of appetite but nothing would induce him to co-operate. The other two bounced round the edge of the hat, their eyes shining in eagerness. No difficulty there. So Saturday passed, then the third day also, and on Monday, feeling distinctly jaded about Monet, I bought a little steak as a change from the lamb. I put a tiny bit under Monet's nose; the effect was instantaneous, and from then on there was no more trouble. All three ate heartily and drank from a teaspoon. Occasionally one would cuff the other and a brawl would ensue. Monet now had a huge appetite and tried to sit on the other two—unsuccessfully, as they were well able to look after themselves. He was the biggest, but so obviously treated as odd man out that I wondered if he was out of the same nest or of the same brood.

Curiosity drove me to Boots. After enquiring at the Prescriptions counter, the assistant who had rescued the house-martins was located at the Pets counter. She was delighted to hear the birds were well and corroborated that she thought there had been two mothers trying to feed the three nestlings which had dropped to the ground after the collapse of the nest or nests. Whether this was actually the case one cannot be sure. When the baby birds had been threatened by cats and boys, their rescuer had taken them into the house and had delivered them to the Veterinary Surgeon next morning, after her unsuccessful visit to the pet-shop.

During the following week Minet, Manet and Monet grew at an astonishing pace. They clustered together (Monet was now more or less admitted) into a lustrous group of gleaming eyes and shimmering plumage, and greeted me by scrabbling out of their basket on to my hand. Soon this scrabbling became a flutter. The inevitable problem arose, when, where and how to release?

Once more I went on pilgrimage to Boots. I was welcomed by the kind assistant and I asked whether she would mind if—when the time was ready—I came to her flat to see where the birds' nest had been and if there were still house-martins around, as it was getting towards migrating time. She was most obliging and gave me her address.

Meanwhile Minet, Manet and Monet had to be put into a

cage as they had started to fly. I allowed them to practise in my room where the lofty ceiling gave them plenty of scope. Now they started to try and fly out of the cage when I fed them. They could fly, but could they feed themselves? Do the two things go together in the case of house-martins? Or does the mother still go on feeding them once they are on the wing?

I rang up Mrs. Marsault. She groaned at the word house-martin, and agreed that the releasing problem was a tricky one. Then she told me that another bird-rescuing friend of hers used to dangle a fly on a thread in front of a problematical house-martin, and if it snapped at the fly, she concluded it was fit to be released and find its own food.

Next morning, being a Sunday, I duly dangled flies. (Anyone who has not tried this would find it a useful addition to the various games of skill usually practised at Halloween parties.) It *seemed* to me that they snapped, but I was terrified of the ever-present mechanism of self-deception and of seeing only what I hoped to see.

They were terrifically lively that Sunday and the Veterinary Surgeon had already communicated to me that he had noted the flocking of house-martins and other signs of their imminent departure. I was caught between the devil of releasing the martins too soon and the deep blue sea of keeping them so long as to endanger their migration.

That evening I visited their kind Boots' rescuer. She showed me exactly where the nest had been. I reconnoitred the area, and found a number of house-martins not far away. Some were still feeding nestlings. I had told the Boots' rescuer that I intended to release the trio the next morning (Monday, 15th September) while the local children were at school, and no-one was likely to notice what was happening.

Accordingly on the Monday morning, accompanied by a very young boy-friend who had been especially interested in their progress and a devoted fly-catcher, I took Minet, Manet and Monet in their cage (after an enormous meal of best steak and bluebottles) to the scene of their release. I opened the car door and opened their cage door. (The cage was on the back seat of the car.) Monet soared into the blue, joining in with other house-martins; he was soon followed by Manet. Minet, bright-eyed, looked around, and just as I was wondering if I ought to take him home for a few more days, he swept out of the car.

That evening I returned to the release spot and patrolled the district. I saw nothing. House-martins were still about.

The next morning the house-martins' Boots' rescuer rang me up to ask if I had released the birds as arranged. I said, yes. She told me she had scoured the area for two hours but had seen nothing. I thanked her warmly and said I, too, had returned to the scene of release. She generously volunteered to patrol the area for a week, which she did. No house-martin in distress was discovered. We can only hope that Minet, Manet and Monet, fortified by steak, are on their way to Africa.

The case of the pitching cuckoo

August 1969. I had not been to my cottage to live in it for a year. At last, after complicated arrangements, attended by frustrations foreseen and unforeseen, I had resolutely turned my back on the College and had arrived at the cottage, complete with Collie, baby hedgehog, sick gull and fledgeling blackbird. 'Now,' I thought, as I settled the gull in the summer-house, the hedgehog in the cellar, and the blackbird in the kitchen, 'I shall have a bit of peace.'

Two days later I went to College to pick up some mail. 'Oh! there you are,' the secretary greeted me with a note of relief in her voice, 'the Veterinary Surgeon has just rung up to say he's got a cuckoo that keeps on falling on its head. Can you go?'

I rang the surgery to find out whether it would be convenient to fetch the cuckoo on my way back to the cottage, foraged for a container suitable for a cuckoo's travelling requirements and went off to the surgery.

Here the Veterinary Surgeon and his wife demonstrated the cuckoo's total lack of balance on the table. 'We don't know whether it's sick or just alcohol,' said the Veterinary Surgeon cheerfully, 'the lady who brought it said she's given it a good dose of brandy—whoops!' The cuckoo had fallen forward on to its beak and seemed quite unable to right itself. 'Says she found it on the ground outside her house,' the Veterinary Surgeon continued, 'and thinks it must have knocked itself out on the window.' 'And alcohol is not the treatment for concussion is it?' I queried, remembering a nightmarish return through the Black Forest with a skier who had concussed himself in a foolhardy attempt at a jump, and who was forbidden a drink at the hotel when we finally reached it. 'I'm afraid not,' said the Veterinary Surgeon. 'Anyhow, tell me what happens. It *may* be that when the brandy's worn off, it'll be different! Perhaps we can tell then.' We put the wobbling cuckoo into the basket-cage I had brought.* 'I think this must be a young bird,' the Veterinary Surgeon remarked as he and his wife waved me off from the door.

'A young bird, and a cuckoo?' I turned this over in my mind as I waited for the traffic lights to go green for the second time, owing to the pedestrians' perverse preference for using the crossing when the lights were against them. What on earth was I going to feed it on? The staple diet of cuckoos was woolly caterpillars; this I knew, and I also knew that ne'er a woolly caterpillar would come my way. Moreover it had probably not come the cuckoo's way either, and that was the likeliest cause of his being a patient—undernourishment owing to lack of caterpillars.

As the cuckoo seemed to like its basket-container I left him in it and placed it on one side of the kitchen table. I put in a flat tray-like basket with a wickerwork edge, thinking that as it was about the size of the cuckoo's body the bird could lie comfortably on the soft tissues I had put in and yet be supported and prevented from pitching by the edges. In order to feed the bird, I followed my usual custom of taking the bird on my knee and when it had relaxed force-feeding it. It swallowed gladly and very quickly perched on the wickerwork edge

* These are excellent containers as they are like a wickerwork tunnel; one end of the tunnel being shut, the other fitted with an openwork wire door. They can, therefore, be used both for travelling and for residence. Birds seem to like them.

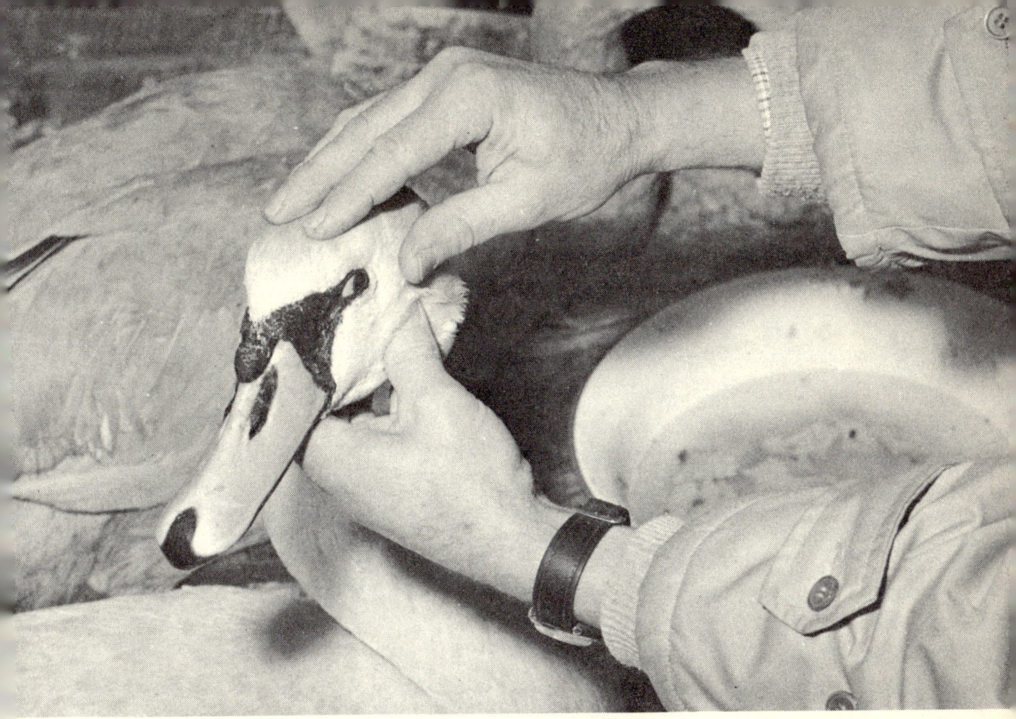

The skilled and gentle hands of the Veterinary Surgeon examining the eye of a rescued swan, blind in one eye.

Famished swans reported in distress at Newhaven. Seen here appeasing their hunger. Note dirty swan on left too weak to stand.

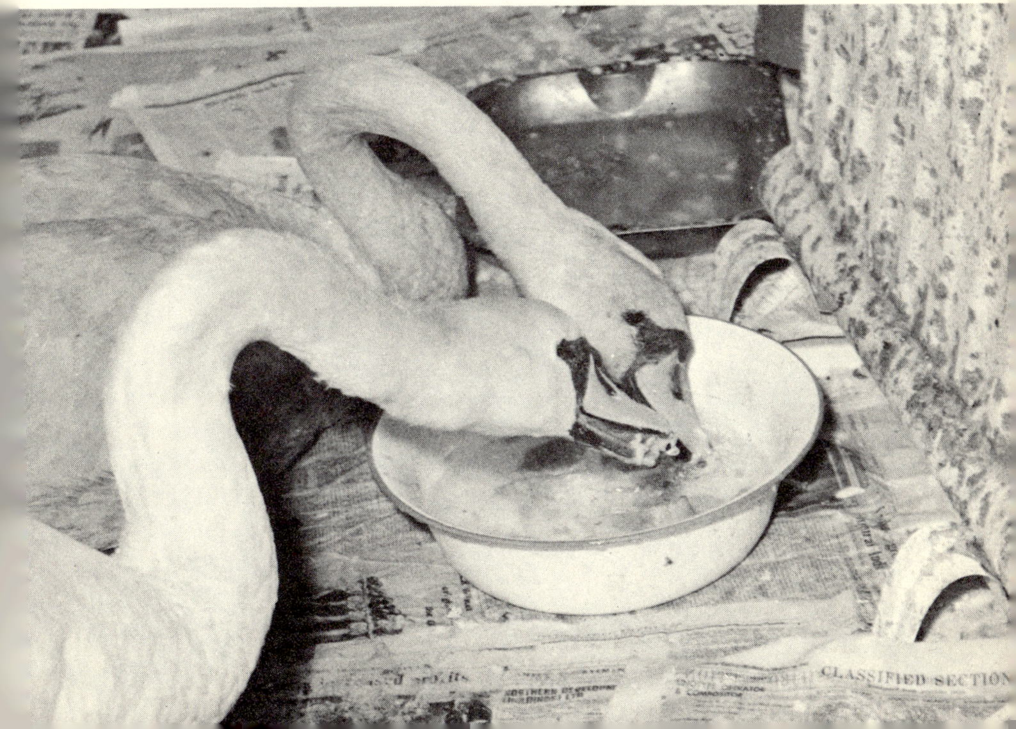

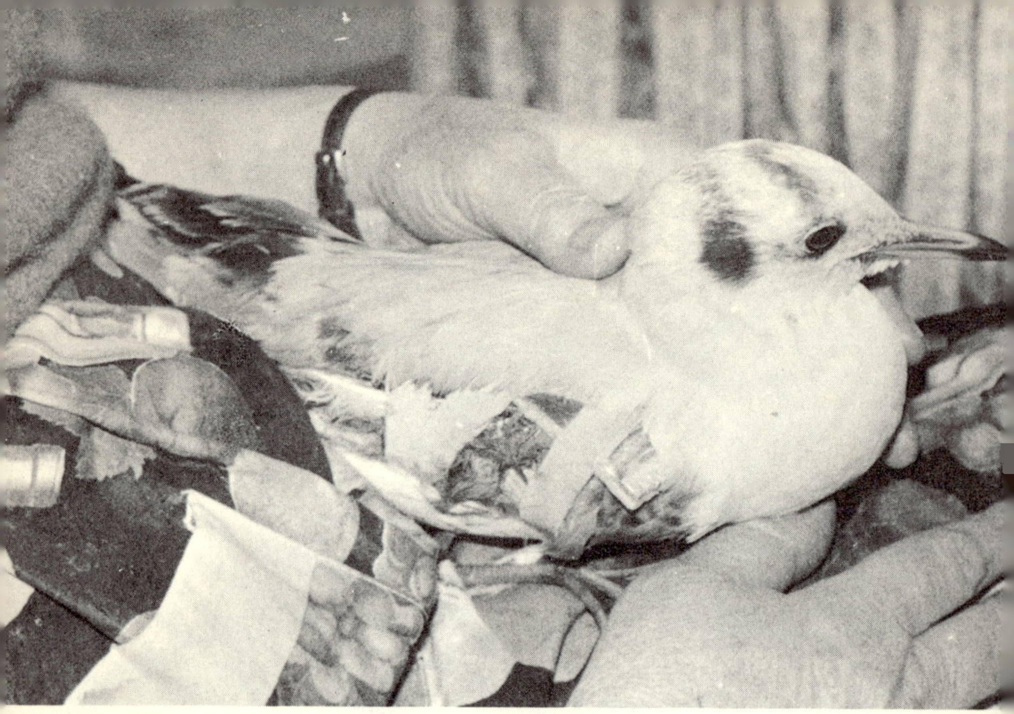

Maynard. Small black-headed gull with badly fractured wing. He lived for 3 months and enjoyed himself. One morning he collapsed and died gently with a trickle of blood from his beak. Post mortem revealed avian tuberculosis.

Great Crested Grebe, found unconscious at level crossing, in very cold weather. Seen here on the road to recovery swimming in my bath.

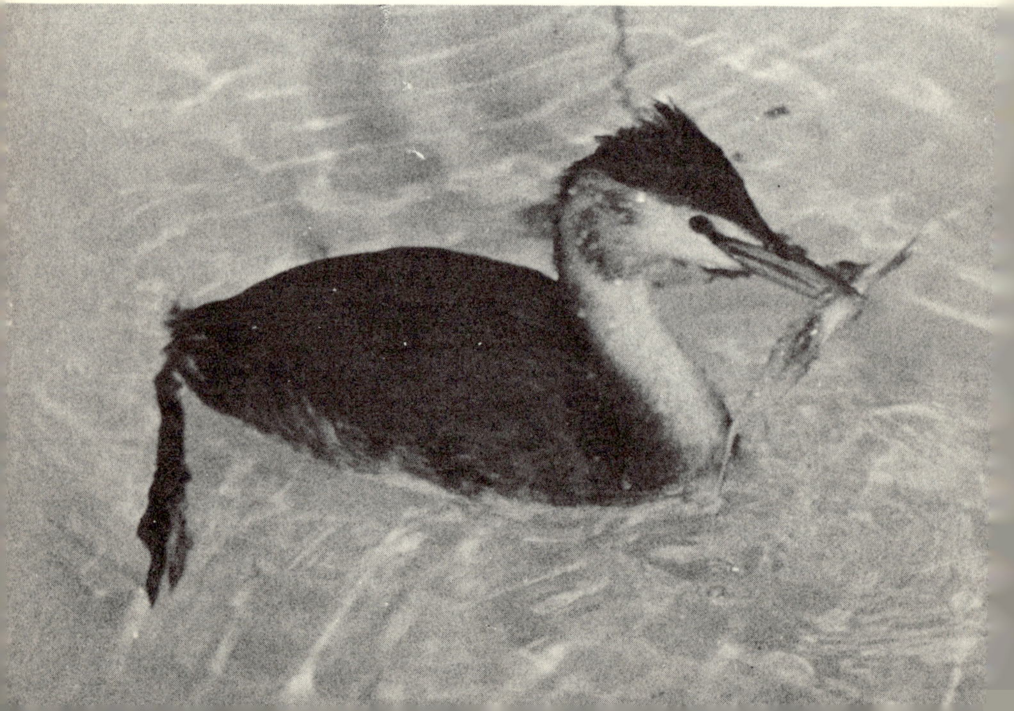

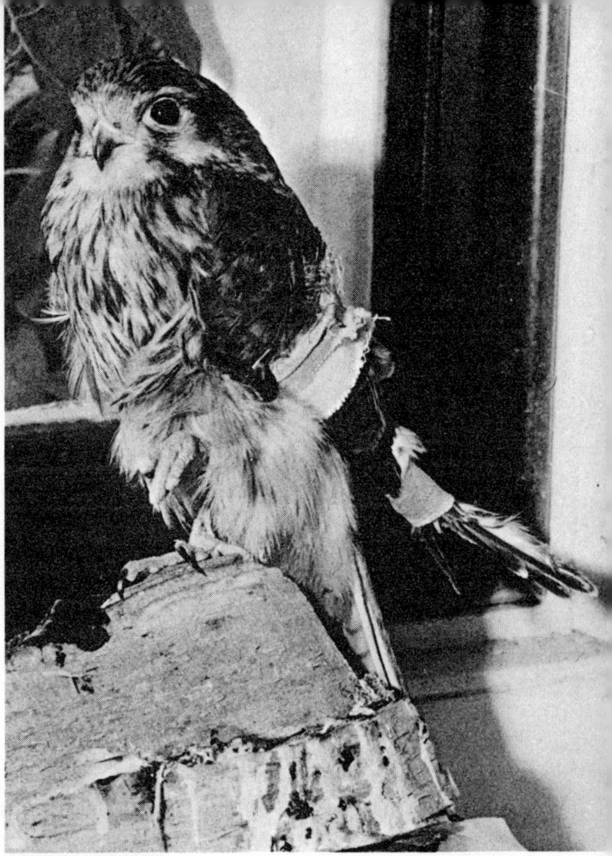

Tiger Tim. Kestrel with smashed-up wing. The V.S. reassembled the wing round a stainless steel darning needle, the only thing small enough. Operation performed under special anaesthetic.

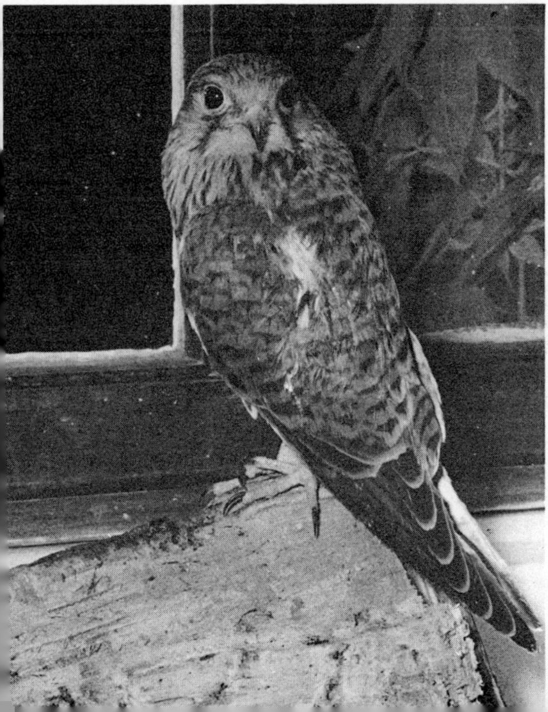

Tiger Tim after his splints and dressings were removed. Note white feathers at the seat of the injury.

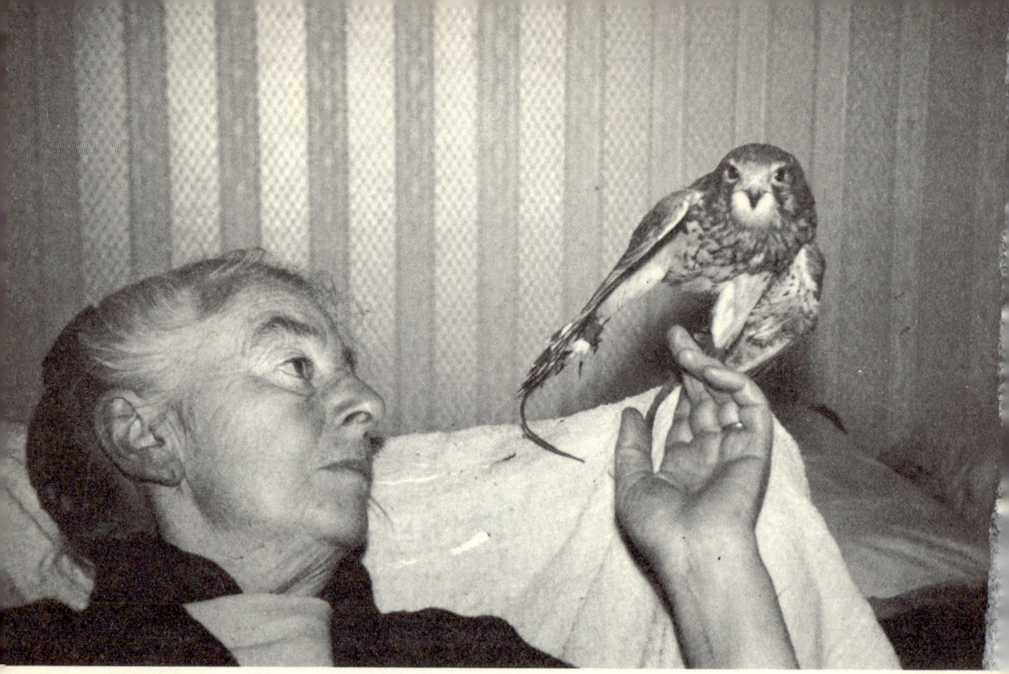

Tiger Tim, on the back of my chair, performing an 'arabesque'. He is wearing jesses only because these may be useful to enable him to be outside in the summer. He now flies a little.

Loopy Loo surprised out of sleep in the fruit bowl by the flash bulb of the photographer. She is onl behind bars by her own choice, as she will only go to sleep in the wooden bowl *inside* a cage, where—on account of her disability—she seems to feel safe. Loopy Loo is apparently suffering from bra damage resulting in a lack of co-ordination, for example she only flies backwards. The damage wa presumably contracted at the time of the accident which caused her to be brought to the surgery witl a fractured leg—now mended. She is a contented, affectionate bird, steadily improving in co-ordination

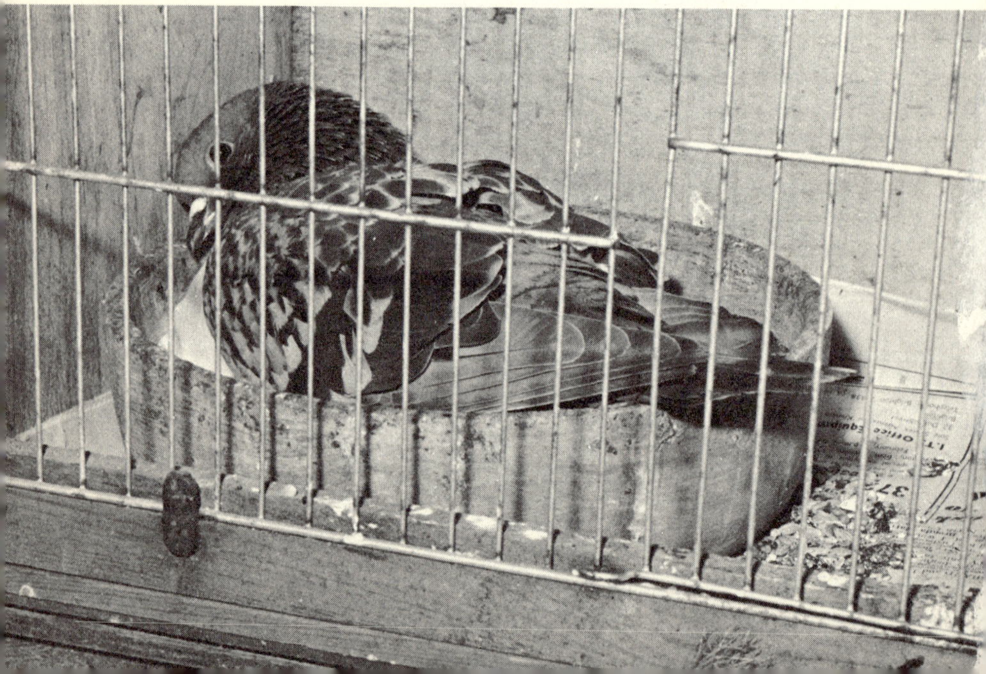

of the basket-tray. This seemed to suit the strange long body, and its claws rapidly increased in gripping power. I also put a little dish of water beside it, but in fact I never saw the cuckoo drink, nor did it show any interest in water.

The first time I force-fed Kuku, the cuckoo ('Kuku' in Swahili means 'hen'), I was amazed to see the brilliant tangerine colour of the whole of the inside of the 'mouth'. It contrasted and yet toned in with the beautiful barred feathers.

The first two days I force-fed Kuku Vitamin B.12 tablets (half a tablet morning and evening) and lamb's liver but on Friday (8th August) I bought some mealworms and steak.

By this time the Vitamin B and food was, I suppose, taking effect and Kuku was much stronger. He started eating mealworms on his own and as soon as I opened his door, he came out, and if I had not already opened the mealworm jar and emptied some on to his little dish, he would tap the jar with his beak. He quickly became extremely tame and when I was indoors I let him roam freely in the kitchen. By Monday, 11th August, he could fly from the top of his basket-cage, where he liked to perch and watch what was going on, to various spots in the kitchen, but did not seem able to 'take off' from the ground. On Monday morning I was feeding him at 7 a.m. when suddenly he looked knowingly towards the open top half of the back door, and without a second's hesitation swept out and into the elder bush at the bottom of the garden. I followed him but he then flew over the neighbour's garden and gaining height disappeared over the roof-tops.

I felt extremely worried on account of his helplessness when grounded. I searched the neighbourhood at intervals during the day but there was no sign of him. At 7 o'clock that evening I was stoking my bonfire in the garden, and as I looked up, I found myself gazing straight into the eyes of Kuku who was sitting a few feet away, perched on the edge of an old copper let into the ground which I keep for liquid manure. He was quite content to be picked up, ate a large supper and went to sleep in his basket-cage.

I have been told that the return of a cuckoo is unprecedented. Whether this is actually so I do not know, but he certainly made himself completely at home after his return, averaging 120-150 meal-worms a day. (I kept up his Vitamin B.12 tablets for about eight days.) His feet increased their grip, and he had ceased to lose his balance. What I did not know was whether he could rise from the ground given the space to do so.

On Friday, 22nd August, a very sunny day, he was itching to fly. I knew if he did not go soon I would have to keep him throughout the winter which would pose its own problems. I considered that on the previous occasion he had voluntarily returned, presumably because he felt himself insufficiently ready to fend for himself. Trusting in his intelligence and the compass in his head, I left the choice to him. He flew on to the top of the tool-shed, then to a lilac bush, and then away over the neighbour's garden.

I told the Veterinary Surgeon with misgivings and the usual doubts as to whether I had done the right thing. 'Yes,' said the V.S. with a mischievous look in his eye, 'I've heard a cuckoo has just been seen flying south over the Eiffel Tower!'

The case of Belinda, the Common Gull

On Saturday, 22nd February, 1969, I received two gulls from the surgery within hours of each other. The first was a black-headed gull and the second a common gull. As I had just been discussing the film of *Johnny Belinda*, the first gull was christened 'Johnny' and the second 'Belinda'. Johnny made a good recovery and was successfully released. Not so Belinda.

Belinda had been taken to the surgery in a cardboard box by a little girl who had found her on the beach and had put her in the box with lumps of haddock. As this had produced no results she had very sensibly taken the bird to the Veterinary Surgeon. The V.S. was out on his rounds and his wife telephoned me immediately. I went to the surgery and when we looked into the box we saw a sad and bedraggled gull, apparently uninjured. When I took Belinda out of her box in the bathroom where Johnny had already made himself at home, she weighed next to nothing and I saw that her droppings were very loose and green. She was too weak to stand and I force-fed her one adexalin capsule and my standard 'mixture' for weak and exhausted birds. This mixture consists of glucose water with Complan added to it. It is an ideal invalid diet and birds which can digest nothing else usually keep it down. On the second day Belinda drank a lot of fresh water, and I continued the adexalin (one capsule per day) and force-fed pipettefuls of the 'mixture' at roughly two-hourly intervals. At the end of the day she could stand and took a few staggering steps. She refused fish, but ate tiny bits of cheese (cheese is beloved by most birds) but vomited some.

I kept daily records, and as I look at these now it is one long battle against Belinda vomiting anything solid that she swallowed. Small worms—about two at a time—stayed down; large ones did not and she then did not even attempt to tackle them. Some bits of cheese stayed down but beyond a certain point they came back half melted. Belinda eagerly ate mealworms but soon vomited these. Finally I stuck to liquid feeds, more or less hourly. This worked, Belinda became much stronger. I had tried mince. Again Belinda ate this eagerly but this was also soon vomited. I began to dose her with Crookes' halibut oil because I wanted her to have something both nutritive and fishy. She liked this and it stayed down. (By this time her droppings were of a normal colour and consistency.) I thought I observed pleasure in her eye whenever she swallowed oil. I reported everything in detail to the Veterinary Surgeon. He suggested a pipette of liquid paraffin. Belinda swallowed this and looked up bright-eyed after her dose. I reported to the Veterinary Surgeon. Still no solids stayed down and it was Friday, 7th March. The Veterinary Surgeon pondered the data and said thoughtfully, 'You know, I wonder sometimes if these birds don't occasionally get an obstruction. After all when you come to think of it, they are voracious; what about a crab's claw or something, getting stuck. Why not try a small dose of castor oil, just a small teaspoonful, and tell me what happens.' I returned to my bathroom and duly administered one teaspoonful of castor oil, floated on glucose water. It was just after lunch and I then took the dog for his stroll. As soon as I got back I went to the bathroom. I opened the door. The floor directly behind the door, where Belinda was wont to lurk, looked as though there had been an explosion; spatters of vomit everywhere—but—in the middle of it all, a large oval weirdly spongy, mustard-coloured solid. Belinda was stalking about looking extremely spry. I collected the solid, cleaned up the mess and offered Belinda some cheese which she ate without the slightest hesitation. Nothing was regurgitated.

I rushed down to the surgery with the 'solid' in a box and left it for the V.S. on his return from his rounds. Meanwhile Belinda ate mince, and a sprat and there was no more vomiting.

That evening the V.S. rang up. 'You know what this is?' he said. 'It's a dahlia tuber. I've just dug one out of the garden and put them side by side, and I really don't think there can be any doubt. Would you care to come down and have a look?' Down to the surgery I went. There was no doubt. No wonder poor Belinda could not get anything past the tuber, and no wonder oil had worked soothingly and had gradually loosened the obstruction. The Veterinary Surgeon cut both tubers in half. They were identical. It was some days before I could get them photographed and by that time Belinda's tuber had shrunk considerably. When first regurgitated it seemed immense. Presumably in her hunger she must have swallowed it perhaps with a worm. At all events she never vomited again. She ate well and developed into a fine bird. She spent the summer in the outside pen. We could not release her at once, as she was not waterproof, but in August she flew off to join the sea-gulls on the golf-course next to the Park. She was a handsome bird, of a patient and appealing disposition.

During her vomiting period she lived on:

Complan, milk and glucose water.
Raw egg (yolk and white mixed) and Crookes' halibut oil (in liquid form).
Adexalin capsules (one a day).
Very finely grated cheese which melted easily.

The case of Mrs. Bates, the Pigeon

The break-bell had just gone when I received a message from the wife of the carpenter working on our College buildings to say that they had found a racing pigeon in the hospital grounds of the hospital where she works. It could not stand and the legs were peculiar.

I went immediately and collected the pigeon. Its legs were peculiar indeed, as they were both badly broken. I took the bird to the surgery after lunch. The V.S. removed the ring and examined the legs very thoroughly. 'You know,' he said, 'I'm not sure whether we ought to keep this bird. There's a double fracture in one leg and a bad fracture in the other.' But the pigeon had already given unequivocal indications of the Schweitzerian 'will-to-live' and I could not help saying, 'Oh! please; do you think it would be possible to try?' The Veterinary Surgeon re-examined everything carefully. 'Very well,' he said, 'leave the bird here, I'll try, and I'll ring you up this evening.'

The following morning I went to collect the pigeon. Both legs were beautifully splinted and Mrs. Bates (as she came to be called, in honour of her rescuer), though very thin, looked happy and comfortable. The V.S. told me that he thought she had been about ten days without food, resting helplessly on her breast-bone.

When I got her home, I propped her up on a hot-water-bottle. She responded well, drank and ate hungrily. I kept her in a cage in my room where I could watch her closely. On the sixth or seventh day she made attempts to stand and flew out of her cage. After that I placed her daily on the rug where she manoeuvred herself around, using her wings as props. After this exercise I put her back into her cage. She was a blissfully contented bird and made rapid progress. As soon as she stood, walked and flew, I put her into my special pen for 'halfway' birds, together with one or two other convalescing pigeons, notably Trousers Ming, a beautiful bird in immaculate white spats. She had been found, sick, dirty and with a badly-damaged wing by a kindly gentleman who had not had the heart to to have her destroyed and took her to the Raystede Rescue Centre in Brighton. Someone said—whether correctly or not I do not know—that she was a 'Chinese' pigeon, hence her name. She remains with us, decorative though not exciting. Her placid temperament, however, has a soothing effect on other pigeons and we use her as a kind of receptionist and hostess.

Weeks passed and from time to time I would remind the Veterinary Surgeon, 'What about Mrs. Bates?' and he would say, 'I'm afraid her legs will drop off!' Actually Mrs. Bates was so much at home in her splints, it almost seemed a pity to remove them. Nevertheless, the day arrived, and holding our breath, Mrs. Bates' legs were unswaddled, and there she stood, upright, with luminous lilac and rose-coloured plumage; slim, strong, and agile. We are all very proud of Mrs. Bates and as a special favour we are allowing her to hatch her first two eggs in the stable.

CHAPTER ELEVEN

Nursing and Learning– A summing up

'But always, as from the very beginning, it was the birds themselves that showed us the way.'
D. Yglesias. *The Cry of a Bird.*

As a very young teacher I once attended a lecture at a large and august teachers' gathering where the speaker was a well-known, and at that time a notoriously heretical educationist. I was one of his most ardent disciples. After a lecture when questions were invited, he took pleasure in making mincemeat of those who asked, admittedly, rather unimaginative questions though they were asked respectfully and in all sincerity; nor was an answer contained in the mincemeat. I vividly remember the hurt of my growing disillusionment as I listened, and the educationist lost one of his most enthusiastic followers that day.

It is not my intention to teach my grandmother to suck eggs, and if some of the observations in this chapter seem pathetically obvious, it is because I have often been asked pathetic—but sincere questions—and a sincere question deserves a sincere answer, not a sneer.

WARMTH

The first priority of any injured or sick bird is warmth. Personally, though I have a hospital cage which can be a god-send for small birds under certain circumstances, I feel happiest with hot-water bottles. I have these in varying sizes, including a number of children's cot-bottles. I collect the discarded woolly vests of students returning to warmer climes than our own, and these make ideal wrappers for hot-water bottles. They are also easy to wash out and dry on the radiator. Moreover the bottle not only provides warmth but is often an ideal propper-up to relieve pressure on an injured part. I have a considerable number of baskets and cardboard boxes of a great variety of shapes, sizes and depths, so that I can quickly pop in a soft lining (old jumpers, pieces of blanket, etc.) and then arrange the bottle or bottles so that the bird can rest at a comfortable angle. I usually put this by the electric fire in my room so that I have the bird under continuous observation. A basket with a handle allows one to drape a towel over three-quarters of the basket without touching the bird, and this keeps them in the semi-dark and gives them a feeling of shelter and security. Sick birds should not be exposed to bright light. (Later when convalescing they may love the sun but should not be over-exposed to it.)

Hot-water bottles must be filled at regular intervals. As I have a reserve of bottles, I simply replace the one on or against which a bird is reclining which ensures the minimum of shifting. If one has to take out a bottle, empty it and refill it and then replace it, it causes much greater discomfort. I find that with a simple replacing system I can usually do this, even when the bird is sleeping, without waking it. Naturally all movements in connection with an ill bird should be of the gentlest.

As a bird recuperates it should never at any stage be suddenly deprived of warmth, nor should it ever be submitted to abrupt changes in temperature. One has again to be guided by the bird and one's own observation to gauge when and how to wean it back to normal temperature. It is better to err on the side of continuing warmth beyond the point where it is essential than to remove it too soon. Nothing is more likely to prevent recovery and to undo weeks of care.

WATER (Drinking)

All birds should have ready and easy access to clean fresh water. The shape and size of the *containing vessel* is important, so also is the level at which it is placed.

The old fable of the fox and the stork still holds good. I once went to the house of a kindly woman who had telephoned me to say she had a sick wild bird. When I arrived she said in crestfallen tones, 'It won't eat or drink anything.' I looked into the small cage where it was temporarily housed. There were two shallow saucers, one with bread-crumbs, the other with water, and as the bird in question had a long neck and beak, I said, 'Could I have a jug of water, please?' When this was brought and held out to the bird at breast level, it stretched its neck, plunged its beak into the water and drank ravenously. 'Well, I never!' said the astonished rescuer, 'I would never have thought of that.'

This lack of what, on the face of it, appears to be common sense is actually very understandable but in view of the bird's suffering, horrifyingly frequent. It does not seem to strike people that it is not a case of 'the bird won't' but of 'the bird can't'. Bowls of varying depths and sizes are on the whole the best containers for drinking water, and if they are heavy, so much the better as they are less likely to upset.

If a bird is immobilised by an injury, the water must be placed so that the bird can drink at will without moving.

WATER (Bathing)

Here the best vessels are, generally speaking, shallow ones, resembling the natural puddles, so beloved of blackbirds and starlings.

When it comes to non-waterproof sea- or fresh-water birds, one has to watch them to see what they require. My non-waterproof gulls love bathing in a shallow dish (about two inches of water and eleven inches in diameter) but they are terrified of anything larger and deeper. They have completely taken over my oval-shaped, enamel chicken casserole which has rings in the base so that they cannot slip. Although I have one of the ready-made ornamental garden pools, they merely walk warily round it, and drink from it. Before I decided on the right bathing-vessel I put down a variety of bowls and dishes, and watched to see which they enjoyed and used most. It is the only way one can find out. In the case of the bathing-vessel one has to consider the material of which it is made. Natural earthenware, being roughish, is very good. I have found birds are wary of plastic containers as they are slippery and treacherous; some birds absolutely refuse to use them; they have my sympathy. One has to remember that if a non-waterproof bird falls into the water, it will drown; and if they are kept in an outside pen, it is necessary to provide a good shelter in case of rain, for when their feathers become drenched they cannot fly either, and are helplessly earthbound.

With sea-birds the question arises of whether it is necessary to supply salt or sea-water. Generally speaking sea-birds drink, and also happily bath, in fresh water, but I always supply *one* bowl of sea-water because I feel they can then drink salt water (which I have seen them do) if they wish, and I always feel the natural sea-water may possibly supply something they need.

SLEEPING

Closely allied to the question of warmth is that of sleep and security. A bird which feels warm and secure can fall into a relaxed sleep, which is as important a healing agent for birds as for human beings. Here again the bird must be watched in order that one may learn his favourite posture, and help him to acquire it if he is prevented by injury or sickness. I often use pads of cotton-wool, and—as already stated—a hot-water bottle to prop up or relieve pressure.

I had an oiled guillemot with a suspected cracked pelvis, and by propping a large hot-water bottle, wrapped in a vest, against the radiator, this formed a soft warm slope. The angle was such that the guillemot could lean against it at an almost upright angle. On his first meeting with it, he immediately sank against it and went to sleep. Later on when the injury was almost healed, he still clung to his angled bottle and became agitated if it was removed even for a few minutes while replacing his sponge-rubber mat by a clean one.

Birds follow what my African schoolboys used to refer to as 'God's time'. They go to bed at sunset and they wake up at sunrise. Hence it is particularly important that they are kept in the dark, or are shrouded, during these hours, to ensure that they get the maximum amount of rest and sleep. At all times a bird should be able to retire into a 'bedroom' so that *privacy* is always available. I am convinced that this is a very important and frequently neglected point. Birds need, and should be able to get, isolated peace and quiet when they feel like it. Some seem to need it more than others, but anyone who has watched birds in their natural environment will have observed them 'resting' alone in some secluded spot. Individual members of even very gregarious birds do this.

FOOD (Variety)

A first experience with a patient of a new species is always unnerving. One knows, or one thinks one knows, what Jackdaws eat, for instance. Experience taught me otherwise. One can look up 'food' in bird-books but this does not get one far. So one tries everything and watches.

I once had two robin fledgelings found abandoned in a stable. The one ate nothing for days but hard-boiled egg and would not touch a worm however small or fetching. The other would only eat worms and cheese, and flicked everything else out of his beak. They both survived and were successfully released. The hard-boiled egg brother for a long while appeared regularly at breakfast time to indulge his preference, and later on, whenever I put morsels of hard-boiled egg on the bird-table a robin promptly materialised in a mysterious way.

In contrast to the example just quoted, birds in general love variety. Again and again, when at last I have found something to tempt a patient's appetite, I have heaved a sigh of relief and thought my worries were over. Not at all. Three days later, or maybe one day only, the titbit recently eagerly awaited with gleaming eye, is inexplicably and stubbornly spurned, and one's food-hunt begins once more. There also seems to be what I can only call 'phasing' in diet. This applies both to sick birds, and where one would expect it, in fledgelings. They have a 'phase' for a certain item of food, and though they may subsequently reject it for a period, they sometimes return to it at a later stage. In the case of fledgelings, however, they naturally grow 'out of' one kind of food and 'into' another.

Quantity. Not knowing how much a bird should eat to keep in good health or even just alive, can be a harassing business. I was frantically worried by my first guillemot, as I had no idea whether it should eat, for example, five sprats a day or thirty. By the time I had nursed several guillemots I had shed at least that worry.

Then maggots! How many maggots make a decent meal for various-sized birds? Only experience reveals the answer, and that is why I have recorded all such answers. I have no doubt others could add different answers, and it is precisely the pooling of knowledge derived from practical experience that is valuable.

RHYTHMS

There is a perpendicular and a horizontal rhythm. The rhythm I think of as 'perpendicular' is the dawn to dusk daily rhythm which resembles a school time-table and can be formulated on a list. The 'horizontal' rhythm is that of the fluctuations over a duration of time as indicated on the 'sprat-charts'. (See Appendix III.)

Perpendicular or daily diet rhythms. When a bird is sick one has to seize any opportunity to get it to eat, and its appetite when ill is often—though by no means always—irregular. 'A little and often' is the usual pattern. As a bird recuperates and reaches convalescence it tends to follow a more noticeably marked rhythm, and may finally settle into a three-times-a-day meals routine. Persistent loss of appetite is ominous and usually indicates the onset of renewed illness or the approach of death, but even so healthy birds have their off-days which need not cause undue alarm. I mention this because I must confess that these 'off days' still tend to cause me disproportionate anxiety.

FORCE-FEEDING AND HAND-FEEDING

It is often necessary to force-feed a sick bird at first, though if one *can* avoid doing it, one should do so. If, however, the bird is so obviously weak or disabled that prompt sustenance is essential, then it is often best to confine oneself to liquid food. Glucose water is a good beginning, or milk and glucose water, and then Complan made up with water rather than milk to avoid being too rich. A drop of Abidec (obtainable at any chemist) can be added. In the case of sea-birds the addition to any of these mixtures of two or three drops of Crookes' halibut oil, goes down well. I usually mix very small quantities so that they do not go sour. I mix a level teaspoonful of Complan, a saltspoonful of glucose to three or four teaspoonsful of water in an egg-cup, and then add the drops of Crookes'. I force-feed the bird either with a small teaspoon or with a pipette. The pipette with the curved end is the best, and one must eject the liquid gently, not squirt it abruptly, and only a few drops at a time or it can go down 'the wrong way' and cause the bird to choke. One must make sure that the bird's tongue is in position, so that the pipette rests on top of it. After use pipettes should be rinsed in hot water. I give a whole pipetteful every hour to largish birds (such as gulls) and two or three drops every half-an-hour to small birds such as blackbirds.

HAND-FEEDING

When one has to force-feed a bird there is often an intermediate stage between that and self-feeding, when it will take food held out to it. In the case of convalescing guillemots I always hand-feed them because then I know exactly what each bird is getting. If a dish of fish is left on the floor, one remains in ignorance as to which bird is eating what, and if indeed one of them is not eating at all. When *force-feeding* a bird I always take it on my lap and let it get comfortable before feeding, but for *hand-feeding* I usually merely hold out the food, or waggle it in what I hope is a mouth-watering manner. As in everything else, there are exceptions to this.

NIGHT FEEDING

As stated in Chapter 2, it is only by being with one's birds at night as well as by day that one really gets to know what is going on.

I had a Great Crested Grebe who used to lie on the hearth-rug like a cat and punctually at 1.30 a.m. and at 4 a.m. he uttered his strange honking cry and clanked his saucer for sprats—and punctually he got them.

Then I found, to my surprise, that the gulls often ate more at night than during the day, though whether they do this in their natural environment, I do not know. I should never have discovered this had they not been living in the bathroom. They used to spend the night standing rather close together (as one often sees them on the beach) and with no tucking in of head. During the dark hours they had active patches when they 'clucked' for food if it had all been eaten.

In the case of a very sick bird one has to use one's discretion as to whether uninterrupted sleep or steadily continued feeding is the more advisable. If I see that such a bird wakes up or has not gone to sleep, I go for the feeding, but if the patient appears to be sleeping quietly and breathing regularly, I leave it in peace and do not wake it. (Would that this principle might be applied in hospitals for human beings!) There is a difference between the healing sort of sleep, and the 'eyes-shut-but-not-real sleep' condition which portends nothing good. One soon becomes familiar with the various symptoms which reveal the true state of affairs, and can act accordingly.

FOOT CARE AND EARTH

If a bird is involved in a long period of convalescence, attention must be paid to foot care, especially in the case of sea- or water-birds, as they are out of their natural element.

Feet get too dry and crack. In the case of guillemots (and similar birds) it is necessary to oil their feet and legs fairly frequently to help to preserve flexibility and to prevent splitting and fraying of the webbing. We first used vaseline. Then, thanks to Mrs. Marsault's recommendation we changed to a cod liver oil ointment, but recently I have turned to Johnson's baby oil and Savlon. The birds seem to find both these preparations soothing.

With gulls I find that the supply of shallow bowls of water for bathing and splashing keeps their feet wet and elastic. Nevertheless, while they are still indoors, I also put down a lare bowl of earth and when not splashing, they spend a lot of time standing on that, whereas the guillemots never take any interest in bowls or trays of sand and seaweed, but stick to their sponge-rubber mats.

With land-birds I also make sure that they have a bowl or scratching-tray of earth (when indoors) and they all make use of it. They also pick up little bits of grit and soil, and they love a scattering of leaves or leaf-mould. Even my monkey is supplied with a dish of fresh earth every day, and apart from playing with it, he not infrequently eats a small lump of earth.

BREATHING, COUGHING, SNEEZING

The way in which a bird breathes is a significant pointer as to the seriousness of its condition. Once a bird starts struggling for breath, gasping, gaping, coughing or sneezing, one must be prepared for the worst, and one should always seek the advice and help of a Veterinary Surgeon. There is a considerable variation in the rate of respiration in birds of different species. In a Great Crested Grebe I counted approximately 14 breaths to the minute as compared to 18 in a human being, whereas I counted 49 in the case of a kestrel. A bird's temperature is 105 to 107 which is why birds do not go septic as readily as human beings, when injured.

I used to think sneezing in a bird was fairly harmless. I said to myself—as in the case of a human being—'he's caught a chill', and duly increased warmth. Alas, the sneezing or coughing patient often died, and recently, in the case of a blackbird, the post mortem revealed 'gape-worm'. There used to be no known effective cure for this, and if a bird shows the unmistakable symptoms it is a matter of urgency to apply the remedy recently discovered by Mr. J. E. Cooper, B.V.Sc., M.R.C.V.S., D.T.V.M., of the Compton Laboratories in Berkshire.* Fatal agony should never be prolonged. Perhaps one day human beings will earn the right to similar mercies.

DROPPINGS

Droppings are also an immediate and easily perceived indication of whether a bird is suffering from some internal trouble. Here, especially, I have felt my own 'not knowing', and am always ringing up Dorothy Yglesias or Mrs. Marsault to enquire what a certain bird's droppings *ought* to look like!

One has often seen the droppings of gulls on the rocks and one's general impression is that they are white. When one lives with a sick or injured gull one is aware of qualities in the droppings not observed before, and realises just how little one knows about such things, and about what is 'normal' in a gull, let alone different kinds of gulls.

Colour, consistency, smell and frequency are the main indicators. The abnormal green of poisoning has already been mentioned. Recently when a guillemot excreted a mustard-yellow excretion, though the bird seemed well, I telephoned Mrs. Marsault who reassured me by saying that occasionally her guillemots too produce these rather alarming droppings, but as the birds continue to progress in spite of this, she has decided that one need not become unduly worried.

Guillemots' droppings, when healthy, are 'squirts', white or watery with fishy, dark-grey, and soft substances in them. A guillemot which hardly excretes or excretes only dry, hardish lumps, usually combined with a poor or non-existent appetite is probably very sick indeed. A recent post mortem revealed

* I am indebted to Mr. and Mrs. John Burkett, authors of *High Fly*, published Pelham Books 1967, for this invaluable information which enabled us to save a kestrel.

advanced aspergillosis (a fungoid and so far incurable disease), the kidneys in this case, being severely attacked.

Other post mortems have revealed avian tuberculosis, ulceration of the intestines (presumably from oil absorption) and aspergillosis. We have also found a peculiarly horrible hard yellow growth in the mouths and throats of owls, rooks and a grebe. Mr. J. E. Cooper has been most generous in carrying out a post mortem for us, and in answering our queries on this subject.

RELEASING

In the un-bird mind releasing a bird seems to conjure up the naïve picture of opening a hand containing a bird and 'letting it fly into freedom'. No picture could be farther from the truth. Releasing a bird which has been a patient, or even a successfully reared fledgeling, is a complicated and nerve-racking business, concerned with 'When? Where? and How?'

TIMING When?

Here, as elsewhere, one can only repeat and warn 'There are no rules.' Nevertheless, for those who, like myself, would gladly pool their findings when confronted with an unpredictable set of circumstances, I would say it is probably better to err on the side of keeping a bird a little longer than necessary rather than releasing it too soon. The latter procedure will almost certainly prove fatal; the former may, but usually does not. Last year I released a sparrow on the early side, as he was strong and seemed so anxious to be off, and I was afraid that further captivity would make him ill. In twenty-four hours he was found dead at my door, and I vowed I would never again take such a risk. I shall keep this vow, though I am aware that I shall be faced with the usual doubts and heart-searching in many, many cases.

In the case of oiled sea-birds releasing presents special problems. To release a rescued sea-bird when it is still not waterproof and, therefore, exposed to certain death—now for the second time—is more cruel than to destroy the bird at once, as soon as it is found. The rescuer of such birds must face realistically what this rescuing means. If the bird survives the de-oiling and shock and escapes the various diseases incumbent upon these conditions, a long period of convalescence and enforced captivity follows which may last as long as twelve months or even longer. The period of re-waterproofing varies with each bird but it will certainly always be a matter of months. A bird is *not* waterproof as long as it gets *wet*. The bird's behaviour is a sure indication of how far from normal it is. At first it will not go near water; as it recovers it will enjoy splashing and sprinkling in a limited fashion. Gradually it may enter a small pool but even then it will not be ready for release. A bird which is ready for release joyfully enters the water and when it emerges, it is completely dry, with no water soaked into its plumage anywhere, the water having flowed off the feathers as it would when poured over any glossy non-absorbent surface.

At present (April 1969) I am receiving a steady stream of sea-birds, mostly guillemots, which appear to have been de-oiled, that is they are clean and white, but which are absolutely non-waterproof and have been found on the beach, terrified. When I get them they eat ravenously, which indicates that they have been wandering on the beach for some time, unable to enter the water and, therefore, starving. Some seem to have picked up oil on the beach; that is they are not covered with the sticky mass of oil as when they have been caught by it at sea but, like dogs on the beach, have a drier oil adhering to their feathers which means they have to be de-oiled again. One guillemot was brought to the surgery by a man who said he had watched it on the beach for three days and had finally managed to catch it. Just exactly how long it had been on the beach is anybody's guess.

WHERE AND HOW?

Having decided that the time has come to return a bird to its natural way of life, the next questions—very interdependent—

to be considered are where? and how? Some birds are territorial birds and if a recently recovered blackbird, let us say, is released on another blackbird's territory especially at mating and nesting times, he may well be involved in a fight ending in injury or death.

For the smaller birds I find it best—if, and when possible—to do a gradual kind of releasing. This depends entirely on one's relationship with the bird and the kind of environment one lives in. If a bird trusts you and still *feels* partly dependent though actually *able* to fend for itself, and you have it in an outside aviary with a door, or half-door, or 'window' which can be left open and which has some sort of alighting ledge on both sides, this greatly facilitates matters. You can leave this aperture open, and the bird can venture out and return at will. Usually the 'return' is regular at first and then becomes erratic till it ceases altogether. Naturally this applies only to the 'ordinary' birds. In the case of Speedy, the swift, for instance, I had perforce to resort to other measures. Once again, it is a case of 'the bird shows the way'.

The difficulty of releasing sea-birds has already been touched upon. Gulls are easier than guillemots. I had a small black-headed gull, perfectly waterproof, suffering as far as we could see from exhaustion and a mild enteritis which after a good recovery, I released on the beach while feeding a flock of its fellows. It took off beautifully and soared straight up and into the flock, where we watched it strongly wheeling amid the others. I returned daily for at least a week at the same time to feed the flock, and to make sure there were no signs of a grounded bird.

I have handed my guillemots to Mrs. Marsault in Exmouth, were I know they are safe, and have received the kind assurance from the Mousehole hospital (now under the auspices of the R.S.P.C.A.) that they would also take on and help me to release any guillemots that were ready to go. In Mousehole the birds are near food and their proper habitat. Every fisherman in the vicinity is acquainted with the Yglesias sisters and the hospital they have seen them build up during the last forty years, and any bird seen to be in distress in the sea is taken there. I would have no qualms about releasing guillemots in Mousehole, still largely free from urbanisation and its influence. There is a wonderful atmosphere about this tiny fishing port, and there is a gentleness about the children in dealing with animals that the visitor can scarcely fail to notice. Wherever the name of Yglesias is mentioned in the village, faces light up, and ever since I have frequented it, I have thought it would be difficult to find a more apt illustration of how the benign influence of sheer goodness in all its simplicity can permeate a community.

THE EMOTIONAL LIFE OF A BIRD AND THE ATTITUDE OF THE 'NURSE' OR 'RESCUER'

What struck me so forcibly in reading Dorothy Yglesias' book *The Cry of a Bird* was that here at last in the writer I had found someone who believed as I did, in the emotional side of a bird's life and character, and who showed an infinitely sensitive understanding of it. In her preface she writes, 'In our belief a somewhat different approach and method* are needed for the deeper understanding of what a bird thinks and feels, which we believe to be possible, though relatively unexplored.' She goes on to suggest that 'many of the actual occurrences described in the book may well bear the construction we place on them, and that, if so, they point to a fuller and more sensitive mental and emotional side to bird character than has generally been accepted.' From my own experiences I was dead certain that Dorothy Yglesias was right, and I felt inexpressible relief at the thought that there were kindred spirits, for, to me, nursing birds and learning from them has always been rather like teaching and learning from one's pupils. Only constant observation illumined by imaginative insight can lead to an understanding of one's pupils' needs, and to solving the problem of how to supply these needs. And so it is with nursing birds.

What has been—in my own eyes—every real failure in teaching has been due to some lack of imaginative sympathy, to some failure to connect the observations and interpret them

* i.e. from 'the normal scientific methods of trained ornithologists'.

to give the right answer, often because one has projected one's own feelings instead of imagining different feelings under a different skin,—and this is precisely the most difficult thing of all, because it deals with emotions.

On the second of my two visits to Joan Hicks* at the Ashington Bird Sanctuary, when she was already ill in bed, I confessed to her that I had—in desperation—nursed Austin Pipper in my hand for five nights. 'That's it,' she said, 'that's what saved him; they *must* be loved.' And indeed mere efficiency is no substitute for love. As a teacher one has experienced the truth of this in human affairs; the warm-hearted, if feckless slum-mother who spanks and loves her brood, is rewarded by the fierce loyalty of her children, while the efficient mother methodically 'treating' her child according to the textbook of psychology is frequently punished by the hostility of a problem child. Equally important is the attitude of the 'nurse' or 'rescuer' of birds. If efficiency is no substitute for love, neither is hygiene. The most efficient 'rescuer' working along irreproachably hygienic lines and surrounded by the most glamorous equipment, is no substitute for love, for love does not work according to theories but is absorbed in learning from the object of the love. I hasten to add this is not meant to be a plea or an excuse for inefficiency or *lack* of hygiene; it is a question of putting first things first and in the sphere of feeling, priority must be given to the emotional attitude of the rescuer. As in all else it is motivation that counts; birds exist in their own right; they are not quaint or amusing 'things' nor yet pieces of property to be owned. Above all they are not experimental material to exercise a rescuer's lust for power. Rescuer and rescued should meet on equal terms.

Birds are intelligent and love company and they easily suffer both from boredom and from loneliness. I do not believe that it is a mere figment of the imagination to say that there are times—especially when they are sick—when birds prefer human company to bird company. They possess an uncanny sense—a kind of spiritual attenae or radar—by which they

* Founder of the Ashington Bird Sanctuary and author of *Their Flight shall continue*. Published J. M. Dent & Son Ltd. 1966.

can pick up the 'aura' of their 'nurse'. I am aware that this will inevitably evoke the scorn and wrath of many of those who advocate and profess a 'scientific' approach. I cannot help it. I only feel certain that Marie Curie, for instance, would have been the first to acknowledge that 'there is more than one way of knowing' (*Hymns in a man's life*. D. H. Lawrence), for she possessed the 'sense of wonder' or as Dr. Schweitzer called it 'reverence for life'.

I have seen different people pick up and handle sick birds, and I have watched the birds' wide variety of reactions, and I hope I have learnt from them.

As soon as a sick bird feels 'safe', it relaxes, sleeps, drinks, eats, or merely rests. It does not move or shrink at one's approach, and there is a curious look of recognition in its eye. This is why I always keep any bird-patient with me in my room, kitchen or bathroom when it first arrives. One must move quietly and unhurriedly, and one should talk to the bird—quietly, of course. One must *live with* one's patients. That is the most important thing of all; that, and always trying to know 'deeper and better and more'.

Useful and basic first-aid equipment for anyone who has rescued a distressed sick or injured bird.

RECEPTACLES—and their linings.

- Baskets of all shapes and sizes. (See photograph.)
- Cardboard boxes of all shapes and sizes.
- Soft felt or woolly hats of all shapes and sizes.
- Wooden bowls lined with soft tissues.
- Babies' soluble nappies. (These make good linings.)
- Soft material, wincyette type, or old jumpers.
  (Make sure the material has no frayed or thready edge, or the bird may get its claws, beak or wings disastrously entangled.)
- Old towels.
- Small hot-water bottles, i.e. babies' cot-bottles.
- Cotton wool.

For a bird with an injury which prevents it from moving or which is too sick to move, the best receptacle is a basket or a box with an old jumper in the bottom, and a baby's hot-water bottle (filled with not too hot water) inside the jumper, with a towel over three-quarters of the top of the basket to keep out the light. This receptacle should be large enough to allow you to put a dish of water and a small tin lid or similar dish of food beside the bird.

Also required—unlimited newspaper.

FRIARS BALSAM—To stop bleeding in an emergency such as that caused by a ripped-off claw. Apply neat to form gluey skin over wound.

ELASTOPLAST STRAPPING—The ½-inch size is the most useful.

DISCARDED ICE-CREAM SPATULAS—These are useful for emergency splints, until a Veterinary Surgeon can attend to the bird professionally.

GLUCOSE or even better GLUCODIN and pipette to administer this—for shock.

COMPLAN—liquid food for exhausted birds, to be hand-fed.

VITAMIN B.12 TABLETS—Usual dose ½ tablet night and morning. ¼ tablet for small birds.

ADEXALIN—Red capsules or in liquid form.

CROOKES' HALIBUT OIL—in liquid form.

The above is a basic list of the most urgently and universally required aids, when a bird has just been rescued.

Always consult a Veterinary Surgeon *as soon as possible.*

CHAPTER TWELVE

The Omega–the Last Word

'And what do your Staff think of all this?' said the V.S. straightening up after attending to a patient in my room. I laughed. 'Oh, they just think I'm a lunatic.' 'The lunatic in the West Wing! That would make a good title!'

'But I'm afraid it would be misleading. People would expect something nice and lurid.'

'All the same, you know, you *should* write all this down.'

I thought about it; perhaps one should. Perhaps one should utter one's cheep; the cheep of a nobody it is true;—the cheep of one of many sparrows uttered in the wilderness.

'You should write this down.' I had heard these words before, many years ago, and just as gently but insistently spoken; on that occasion by the late Sir Herbert Read. Strewn around us on tables and chairs in the Centre for Industrial Design lay paintings by children in Africa which I had brought with me on leave in the hope that *someone* would understand, and how marvellously my prayer had been granted.

Curiously enough it was a kind of parallel. Teaching is an art, but in these days of battery pupils and students, it is difficult to make oneself understood, for inevitably the artist's approach is one of humility in the face of his awe-inspiring material. My pupils have been my teachers. It is the same with birds—teachers of my childhood.

Nor have the heroes of my youth lost their stature. Dr. Albert Schweitzer still heads the list, and his message 'Reverence for life' has merely gained through the passage of time; gained in significance and in its terrible urgency. And in the end that will remain the last word—reverence—reverence for all that lives, and without reverence and wonder there can be no love.

Never has the prophetic message clothed in the magnificent imagery and cadences of the letter to the Corinthians been more pertinent than now in this clever age; for truly, though we speak with the tongues of men and of angels, and have not love, we are become as sounding brass, or a tinkling cymbal. And though we have the gift of prophecy, and understand all mysteries, and all knowledge . . . and have not love, we are nothing . . . . Whether there be prophecies, they shall fail; and whether there be tongues, they shall cease; whether there be knowledge, it shall vanish away;—for now we see through a glass, darkly—and there abide, faith, hope, love, these three; but the greatest of these is love.

APPENDIX I

Jackie Whiskers' (Jackdaw) diet sheet.

Maggot pupae (would eat up to 80 at one go!).
Mealworms (2 or 3 at a time).
Hard-boiled yolk of egg. (⅓ or ½ of a teaspoonful at a time).
½ a glacé cherry.
1 or 1½ raspberries. (Perhaps 2 or 3 times a day).
Flies (singly with other things).
A few woodlice.
A spot of cooked fish.
A small lump of fruit cake. (He did *not* like bread).
A sultana or two.
A little squashed peanut.
A little 'Lassie' dog food.

He would not touch meat of any kind, which is often the case with the insectivorous/fruitarian birds.

APPENDIX II

Two days' mealcharts for Speedy, the swift.

Wednesday, 31st July.

5.30 a.m.	3 bits steak. 1 sip glucose water.
6.30 a.m.	1 bit steak.
6.50 a.m.	1 bit steak.
7.45 a.m.	Glucose water.
8.20 a.m.	3 flies soaked in liquid adexalin. 1 teeny steak.
9.30 a.m.	1 bit steak.
9.50 a.m.	1 bit steak.
10.00 a.m.	3 flies.
10.30 a.m.	(after eye swabbing) 2 bits steak.
11.00 a.m.	1 bit steak.
11.40 a.m.	2 flies.
12.10 p.m.	1 bit steak.
1.00 p.m.	1 daddy-long-legs.
1.50 p.m.	1 mealworm larvae. 1 bit steak.
2.20 p.m.	1 fly.
3.30 p.m.	1 bit steak.
4.50 p.m.	1 fly. 1 bit steak.
5.50 p.m.	1 bit steak.
6.20 p.m.	1 bit steak.
10.30 p.m.	1 fly. 1 bit steak.
Total	18 bits steak.
	11 flies.
	1 daddy-long-legs.
	1 mealworm larvae.
	Glucose water (he had more of this than actually recorded as I offered it now and again, and also sometimes dipped the steak in it, but only *slightly*. I did *not* give sodden or runny snippets).

Thursday, 1st August

7.00 a.m.	2 bits steak.
8.00 a.m.	1 fly. 1 bit steak.
8.45 a.m.	1 bit steak.
9.40 a.m.	2 flies in adexalin. 1 bit steak.
10.10 a.m.	2 bits steak.
11.10 a.m.	2 bits steak.
11.30 a.m.	1 bit steak.
11.35 a.m.	1 large bit steak.
1.30 p.m.	2 bits steak. 1 fly. Glucose water.
2.00 p.m.	2 flies. 1 bit steak.
2.30 p.m.	2 bits steak.
3.30 p.m.	2 bits steak 'garni' i.e. rolled in greenfly.
4.05 p.m.	2 bits steak in greenfly.
4.40 p.m.	3 bits steak in greenfly. (Speedy had soon regis-stered this as a delicacy!)
8.00 p.m.	2 bits steak in greenfly.
8.20 p.m.	2 bits steak.
Total	27 bits steak (and greenfly).
	6 flies.
	Glucose water.

The times may seem erratic but they were determined by a) my teaching timetable and b) Speedy's own reactions. He was, on the whole, sleepy in the afternoons, liked a good feeding programme till he went to bed, so to speak. Here, as already mentioned, my excursions into the bathroom might rouse him, and whenever he twittered energetically, I always fed him.

APPENDIX III

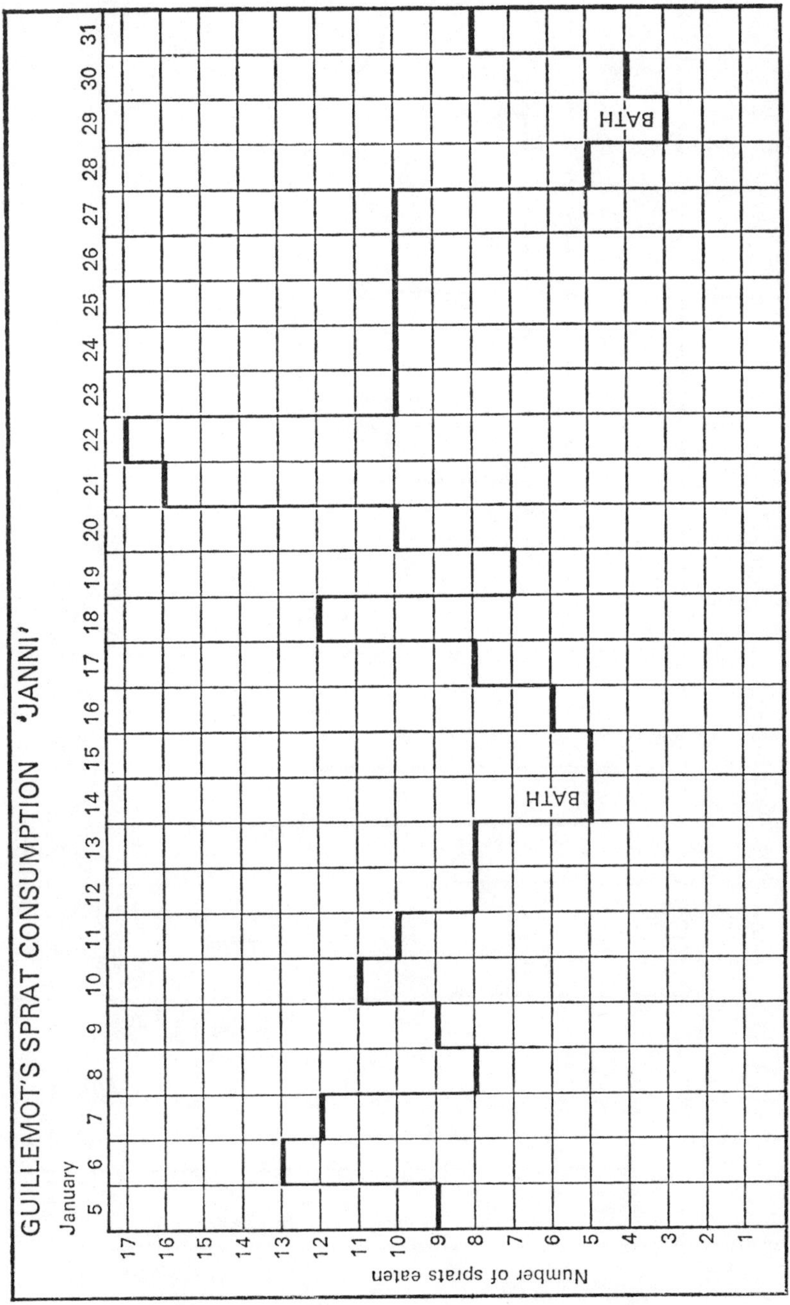

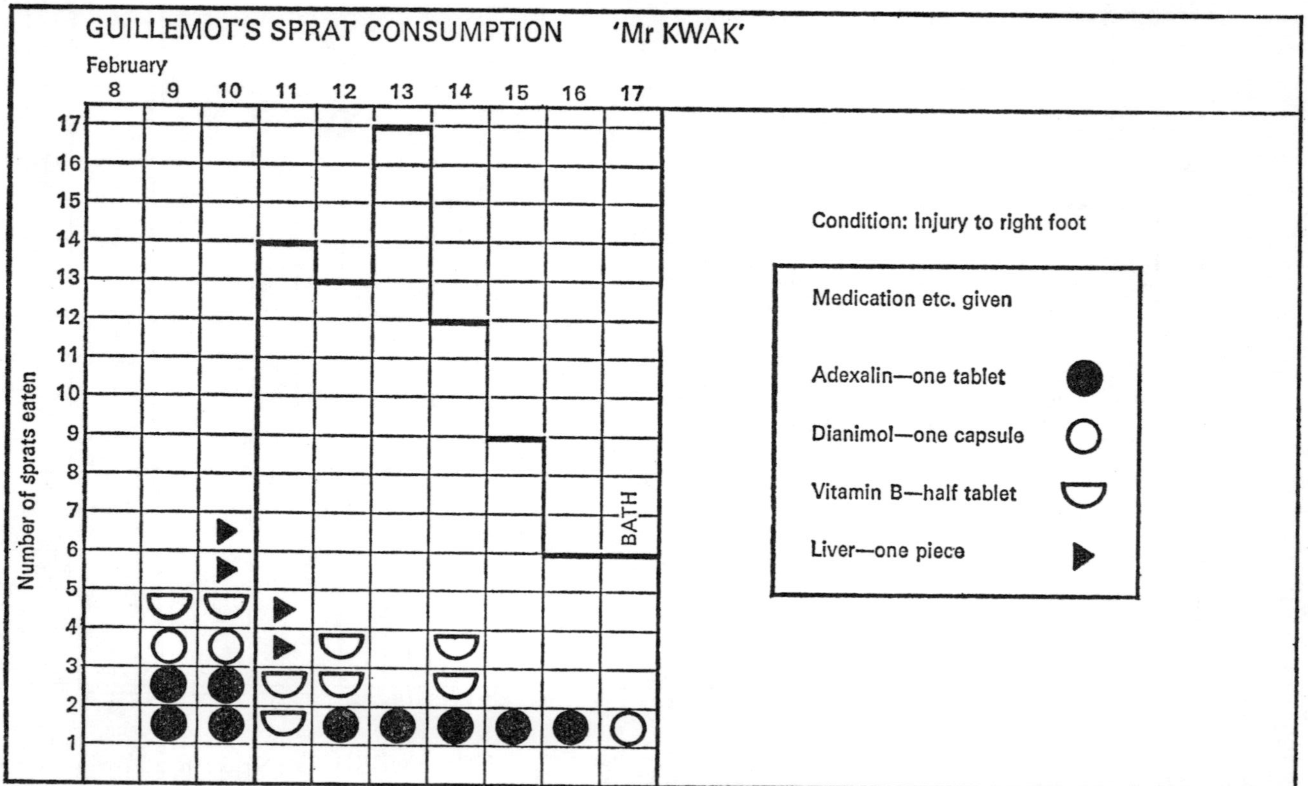
GUILLEMOT'S SPRAT CONSUMPTION 'Mr KWAK'
February
8 9 10 11 12 13 14 15 16 17
Number of sprats eaten
17 16 15 14 13 12 11 10 9 8 7 6 5 4 3 2 1
BATH
Condition: Injury to right foot
Medication etc. given
Adexalin—one tablet
Dianimol—one capsule
Vitamin B—half tablet
Liver—one piece

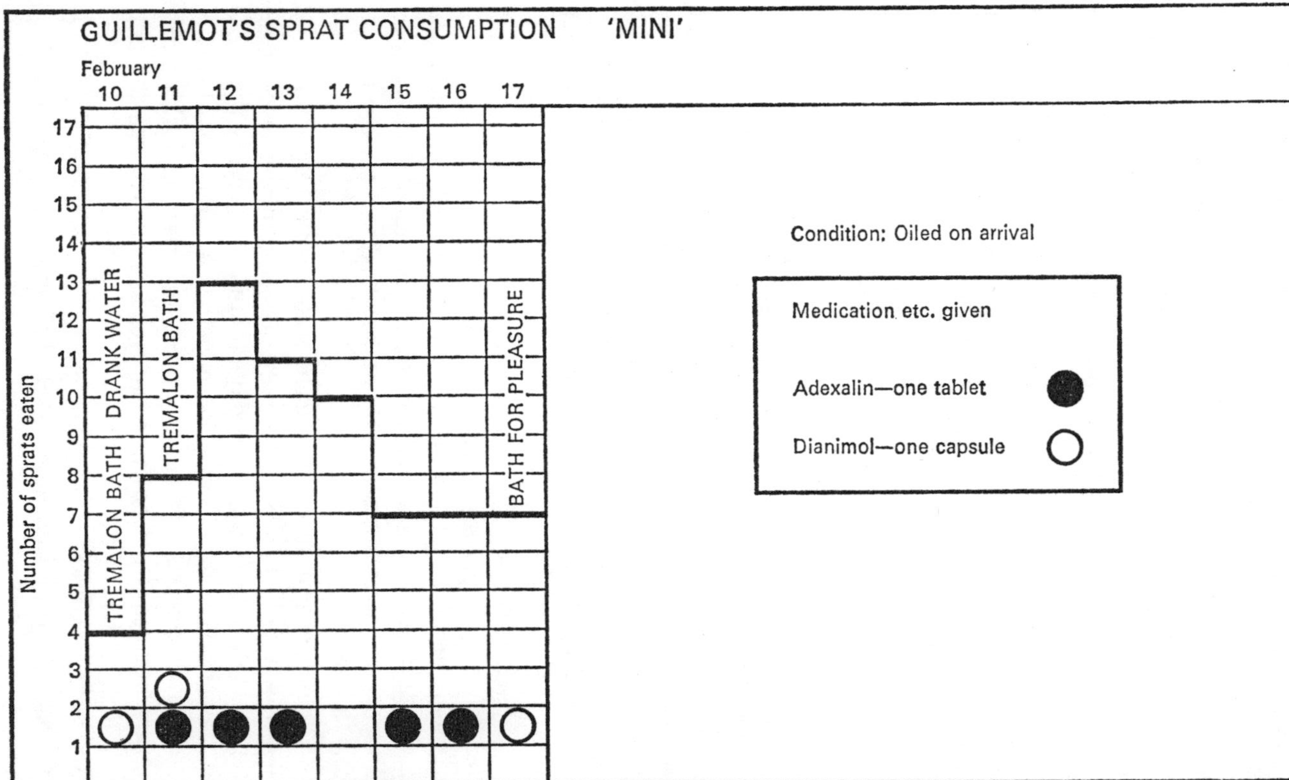

GUILLEMOT'S SPRAT CONSUMPTION 'MINI'
February
10
11
12
13
14
15
16
17
Number of sprats eaten
17
16
15
14
13
12
11
10
9
8
7
6
5
4
3
2
1
TREMALON BATH
DRANK WATER
TREMALON BATH
BATH FOR PLEASURE
Condition: Oiled on arrival
Medication etc. given
Adexalin—one tablet
Dianimol—one capsule

APPENDIX IV

Daily diet sheet for Binkie, the blackbird, as in February, 1969.

On waking Binkie sings, and will sometimes eat a few maggots, at about 7 a.m. (If too busy singing he won't!).

Then I put down his real breakfast which is a bowl of fresh earth (important) and on top:

A dessertspoonful of Swoop.

A teaspoonful of uncooked porridge oats.

Some chopped apple (half a teaspoonful).

3 sultanas or raisins.

Some chopped Cheddar cheese (half a teaspoonful).

(Binkie prefers Danish Blue but I often have forgotten to get it!)

Some ants' eggs (obtainable in pet shops).

At 11 a.m. I give him some meal-worms (about 6) or a teaspoonful of chopped lean lamb (raw).

At 1 p.m. some maggots (about 5) and a little brown bread soaked in milk (or broken digestive biscuit).

At teatime, some cornflakes and perhaps more cheese or an earthworm or two from the garden. (Binkie is not keen on worms. He adores blue-bottles and any kind of caterpillars or grub, and *slugs.*)

Supper 6.30 p.m. Same as breakfast but with at least a full teaspoon of chopped lean lamb (raw).

Sometimes I give lamb at midday too depending on Binkie's appetite. I vary these ingredients naturally i.e. sometimes I give an extra lot of meal-worms and no cornflakes or more sultanas, and so forth.

One curious thing remains to be recorded in connection with Binkie's feeding habits. Even now, as an adult he likes to be hand-fed once or twice in the day, and most especially at night. If I am busy or am delayed he mopes. It is difficult to explain what this consists of, but he takes up his 'mopish' stance, rather huddled, head down, with eyes looking up, and if I put my hand down in his vicinity he often gives me a sharp peck first before eating as though to punish me, whereas if I arrive at the right time I do not receive this severe reprimand.